Fat Loss Secrets:

What Works, What Doesn't

*An Interactive Workbook
for Easy Diet and Activity Analysis
to Achieve Quick & Lasting Results*

by

Lily Splane, M.N.

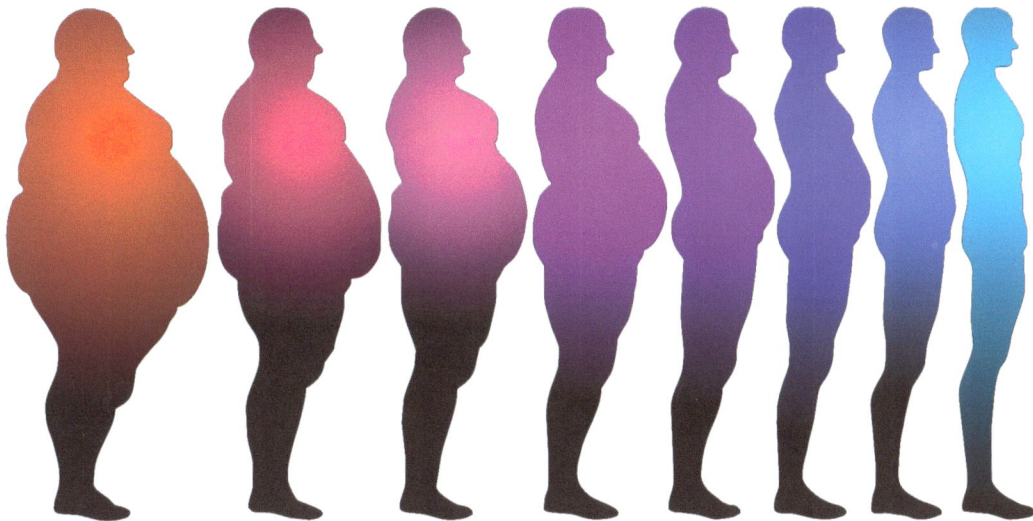

Anaphase Publishing
A Division & Imprint of Cyberlepsy Media
San Diego, CA
www.Cyberlepsy.com

Fat Loss Secrets:
What Works, What Doesn't

An Interactive Workbook
for Easy Diet and Activity Analysis
to Achieve Quick & Lasting Results

Portions of this book have been excerpted from
Nutritional Self-Defense: Better Health in a Polluted, Over-Processed, and Stressful World,
by Lily Splane, M.N.
published by Anaphase II Publishing, 2003, ISBN 13: 978-0-945962-13-7

ISBN 10: 0-945962-48-7
ISBN 13: 978-0-945962-48-9

Published and Printed in the United States of America

by

Anaphase Publishing
A DIVISION & IMPRINT OF CYBERLEPSY MEDIA
4669 Cherokee Avenue, Suite E
San Diego, CA 92116-3654
WWW.CYBERLEPSY.COM

Table of Contents

Preface..7

Introduction..9

Natural "Real" Foods..11

Processed (Manufactured) Foods......................................14

   The Conspiracy 16

HEALTH CONCEPT #1...17

   Your Body's Energy Balance 17

      Energy Input 18

      Energy Output..21

         What Governs Biological Energy Transformations? 21

HEALTH CONCEPT #2...24

   Calories from Macro-Nutrients 24

      Instructions...24

   Your 24-Hour Food Journal..25

      Self-Assessment 26

HEALTH CONCEPT #3...27

   Macro-Nutrients in Food..27

   Carbohydrates..27

      The Saccharides (sugars & starches) 29

   Fiber: The Indigestible Carbohydrate 31

      Compounds Produced when Fiber Intake is Inadequate 32

      Instructions...32

      Self-Assessment 35

   Modern Grains: The Staff of Life...? 35

      History of Grains 35

      Modern Wheat...37

      Health Effects of a High-Wheat Diet 38

      Blood Sugar and Insulin..38

      High Wheat Intake and Lipidemia (High Blood Fats).................39

      Body pH and Wheat..39

      Gluten, Gliadin, and Lectin.......................................40

      Moving Forward...40

    Corn..41

    Rice..44

  Protein..46

    Protein Quality 46

    Combining Foods to Complement Amino Acids 48

      The "Limiting" Amino Acids (LAA) 48

      Instructions...49

      Instructions 59
      Self-Assessment 60
  Protein Deficiency Diseases 61
Dietary Fats (Lipids) 61
  Unsaturated Fat (Triglyceride) Molecule 61
  Saturated Fat (Triglyceride) Molecule 61
  Unsaturated Fat (Triglyceride) Molecule 62
  Saturated Fat (Triglyceride) Molecule 62
  Bad Lipids 63
  Good Lipids 64
      Polyunsaturated Fatty Acids 64
      Omega-3 Fatty Acids 65
      Monounsaturated Fatty Acids (Omega-9s) 65
      Saturated Fatty Acids 65
      Tropical Oils 66
      Dairy Fats (butterfat) 67
      Conclusion 68
  Ratios of Saturated, Polyunsaturated, and Monounsaturated Fats 69
      Instructions 69
      Self-Assessment 72

HEALTH CONCEPT #4 ....**73**
Processed Food 73
  Assess Your Processed Food Intake 73
      Instructions 73
      Instructions 75
      Self-Assessment 76

HEALTH CONCEPT #5 ....**77**
Dieting Strategies 77
  Dubious "Fad" Diets 77
      Low-Calorie Diet (Weight Watchers, etc.) 77
      One-Food-A-Day Diet 78
      Special Prepared Meals (Jenny Craig, etc.) 78
      Eliminating Food "Villains" 79
      High Protein, Low Carbohydrate Diet (Atkin's, Ketogenic) 79
      Water-Loading Diet 80
      Liquid Protein Diet (Protein-Sparing) 81
      Herbal Powder Diets (Herbalife, etc.) 81
      Fruit-Loading Diet (Beverly Hills or Hollywood Diets) 81
      HCG Injections (Human Chorionic Gonadotropin shots) 82
The Most Important Concept You'll Ever Learn:
Insulin, Hyperinsulinism, and Inflammation ***82***
  Insulin-Glucagon Axis
  and Eicosanoid Pathways 83

Glycemic Index and Glycemic Load 86
Calculating Glycemic Load 87
    Instructions.. 94
    Self-Assessment 96

HEALTH CONCEPT #6 98
Energy Expenditure During Daily Activities.............................. 98
How to Calculate Your BMR (Basal Metabolic Rate) 98
    METHOD 1: A General Calculation................................... 98
    METHOD 2: Precise Energy Requirement Calculation......... 99

HEALTH CONCEPT #7 106
Exercise for Weight Control 106
Hazards of Endurance and "Cardio" Training 106
Exercise Physiology and Benefits of
High-Intensity Interval Training (HIIT) 107
    Assessing Your Fitness Level 109
    Instructions.. 109
    Self-Assessment 109
    Finding Your Recovery Heart Rate 110
    Instructions.. 110
    Self-Assessment 110
Interval Training Routines 111
    Instructions.. 111
    Sample Interval Training Routine 112
    UNFIT LEVEL Interval Training Routine 112
    Sample Interval Training Regimen for GENERALLY FIT Persons........................... 112

HEALTH CONCEPT #8 113
Micro-Nutrients: Vitamins, Minerals, and Enzymes 113
Nutrient Chirality (Polarity) 114
Enzymes 115
Preparing Foods... 115
    Produce.. 115
    Breads, Meats, and Root Vegetables 116
    Grilling and Barbecuing.. 116
    Eggs 117
    Fats in Baking... 117
Summary.. 117

APPENDIX
Nutrition Tables.. 118
    Standard Serving Sizes 118
Supplements That Lower Blood Glucose 135
Recommended YouTube Videos on Nutrition and Endocrinology 137
References 138

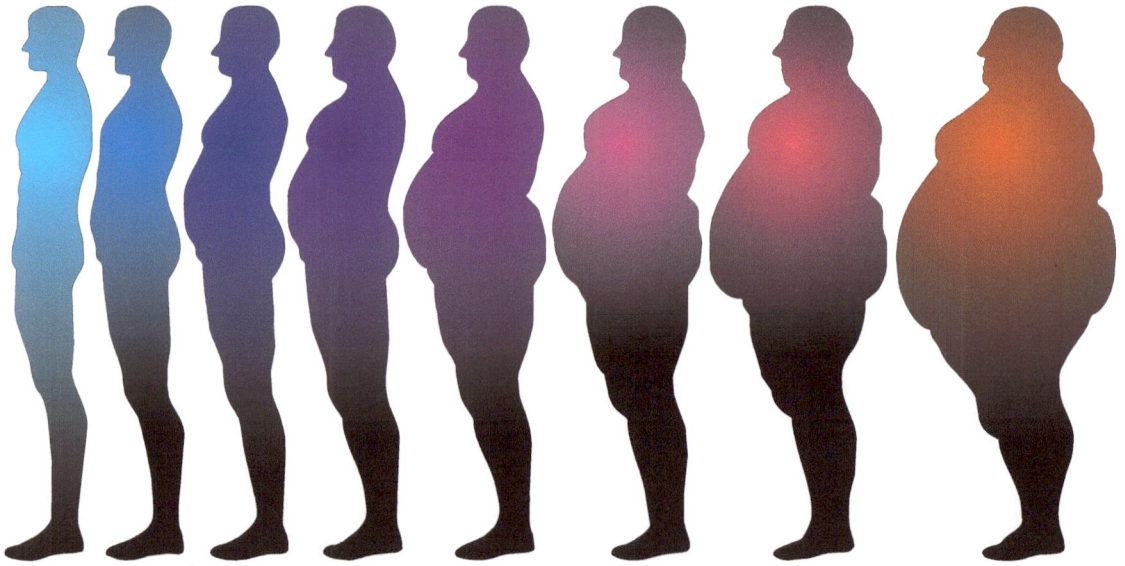

Preface

This book is for people who don't like to read research on diet and exercise, trying to figure out what might work and what might be bogus. Contained herein is the current information you will need to ease into a lifestyle of better health and well-being. There are no recipes or bizarre programs to follow. It's all really a matter of living with your inherited physiology, rather than trying to design a lifestyle that requires you to study volumes of nutrition and exercise books, trying to find a "fit" you can live with.

This approach to good health will work for anyone of any age, physical condition, or food aversions (or obsessions!). There are only two principles to understand: They are straightforward and uncomplicated, and completely adaptable to your preferences.

1. Your diet should consist of mostly plants, with lean meats, nuts and seeds, and dairy products as sources of important nutrients. *That's it.*

2. You'll discover that a mere 15 minutes daily of exercise is all that is required to get fit and stay that way for life.

As you learn in each of 8 *Health Concepts* chapters, you will be invited to engage in the analysis of your own health—as it now stands—with self-assessment questions and activities, permitting insight into your status and goals.

Get ready to become your favorite subject of study!

Lily Splane, M.N
San Diego, October, 2014

Introduction

"Education consists of what we have unlearned."—Mark Twain

Worldwide, no diet quite compares with that of the United States. Though we enjoy the most varied availability of foods in the world, pound for pound, processed pseudo-foods far outsell fresh vegetables and fruits. As a consequence of our industrialized, processed food supply, the United States suffers from the most diet-based disease in the world, which includes metabolic syndrome (a pre-diabetes condition presenting with a constellation of symptoms that includes easy weight gain, high blood pressure, blood sugar irregularities, high triglycerides, and high cholesterol), type-2 diabetes, heart disease, cancer, and even arthritis. All of the aforementioned chronic diseases can be prevented and even improved with diet and minimal exercise.

Humans are not biologically designed for consistent "rich" (processed and refined) food intake. We are still very much physically adapted to the active hunter-gatherer lifestyle of the African Savannah of 100,000 years ago. Yet, we live in a strange new world of our own creation that deviates considerably from the requirements of our own ancient physiology.

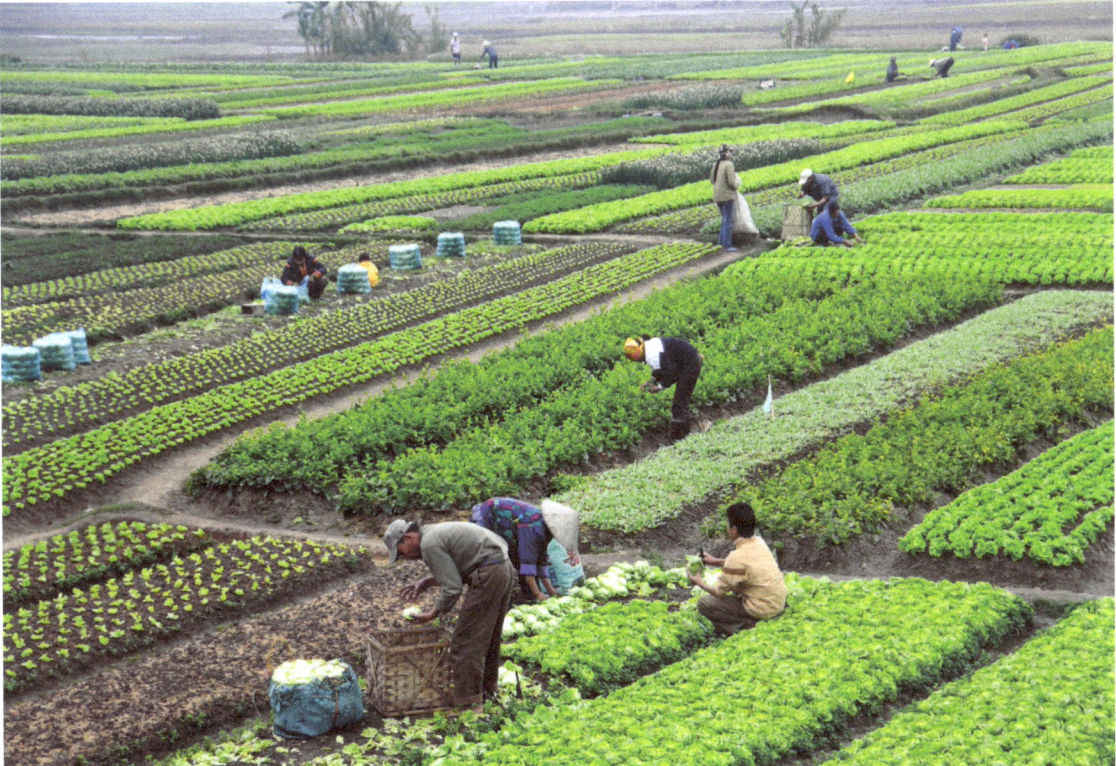

Agriculture through manual labor was the predominat cultivating technique of the past.

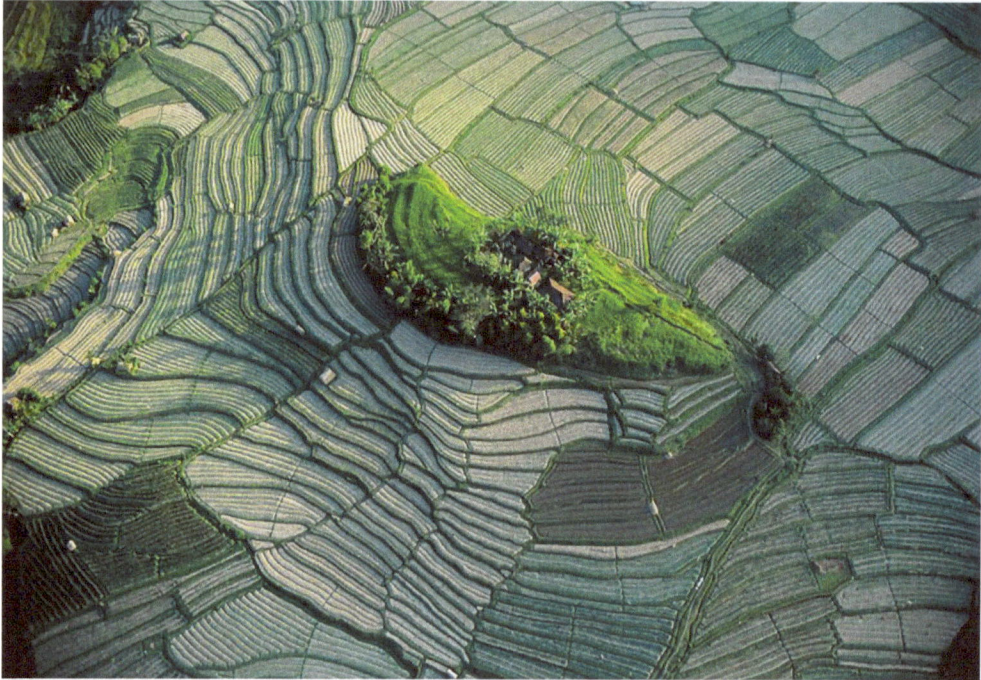

Traditional rice terrace cultivation is thousands of years old and still practiced today in rural China and other far-eastern countries.

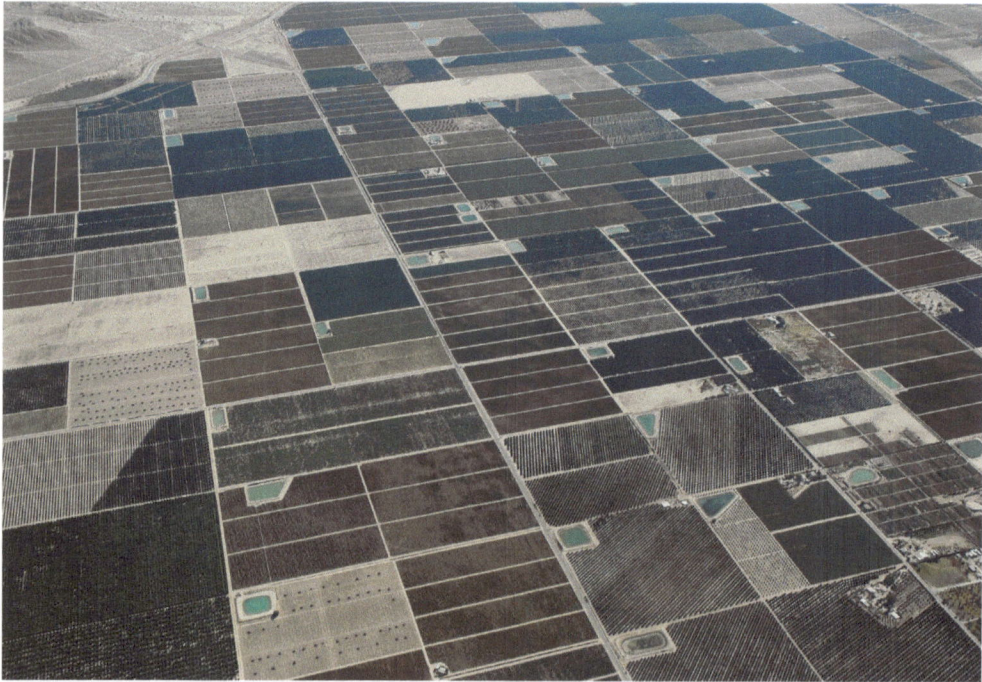

Coachella Valley, CA. Modern agriculture occupies thousands of acres, growing the same crops in the same area year after year, depleting the soil of minerals, which are replaced with synthetics.

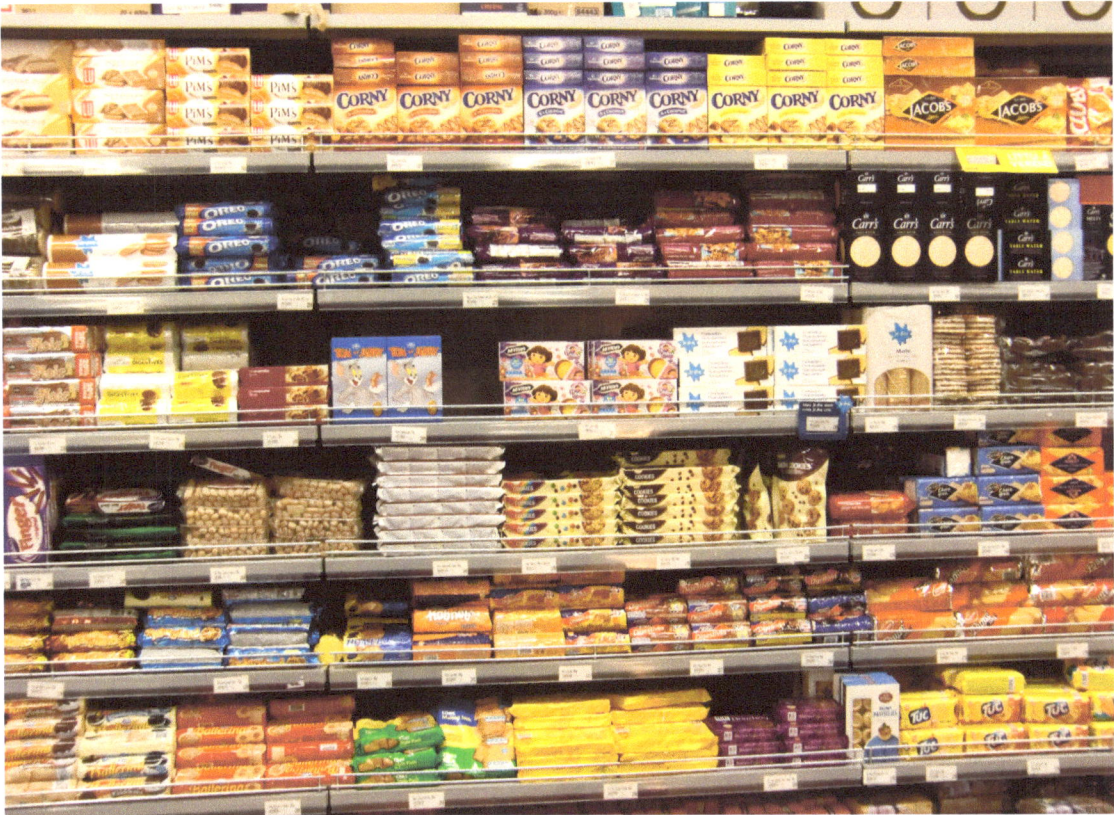

Today, modern humans gather and consume packaged processed food from a market, jeopardizing health.

Better health entails getting back to our ancient foundations: the foods we ate, and the way we have exercised for eons. Better health means becoming more attuned to how we feel (and what our blood tests indicate) when we deviate from our natural roots, and making subtle changes that will build and maintain optimally functioning bodies.

Natural "Real" Foods

The foundation of a healthful diet is unprocessed food consisting of mostly plants. Many decades of research throughout the world have confirmed the value of a plant-based diet complemented with lean protein sources and fruit- and nut-based (olive, avocado, walnut, coconut) dietary oils. The addition of nuts, seeds, and modest amounts of whole-grain–based foods provides additional fiber and nutrients. Examples of this kind of diet may be found in most Mediterranean countries, the Middle- and Near-East, parts of Africa and South America, India, and rural China.

Natural, unprocessed food provides significant nutrients such as vitamins, minerals, and enzymes absent from commercially processed food. In addition to those nutrients, natural plant-based food supplies fiber which is necessary for proper digestion, blood sugar control, and attaches to excess dietary fats to reduce their absorption.

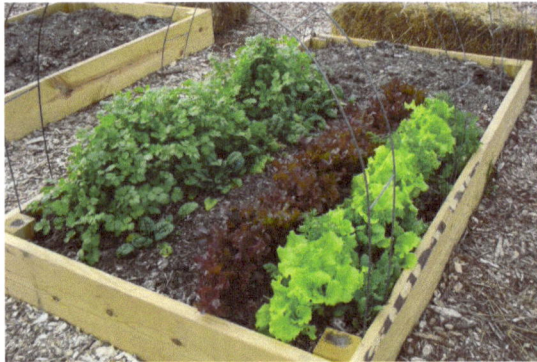

Natural, raw foods are more healthful than processed foods, and contain vitamins, minerals, and phyto-enzymes not found in processed foods.

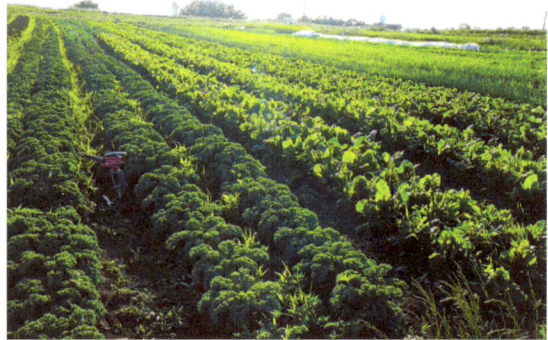

Even commercially grown produce is vastly superior to the packaged processed "pseudo-foods" found on supermarket shelves.

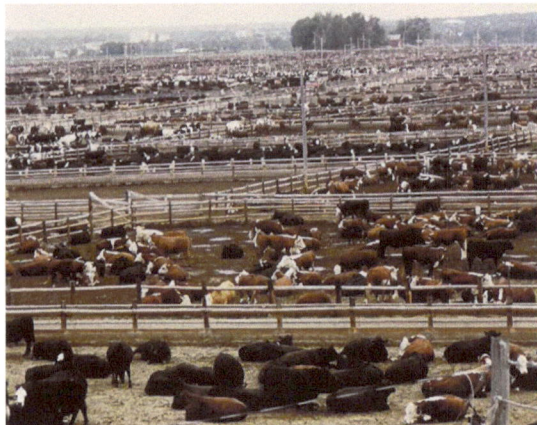

Modern beef raising practices include enclosing thousands of animals in CAFOs—Confined Animal Feeding Operations—where they are overfed on grain to fatten them and increase meat marbelization.

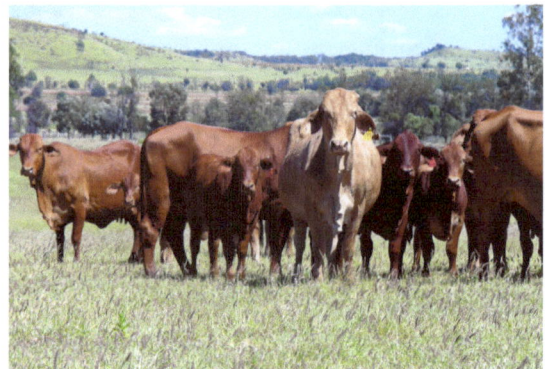

Grass-fed cattle allowed to graze naturally year-round create beef that is leaner and higher in omega-3 fatty acids, and low in inflammation-causing fats.

Nebraska has the highest concentration of CAFOs of any state in the Union. Each dot in this graphic represents at least 500 cattle.

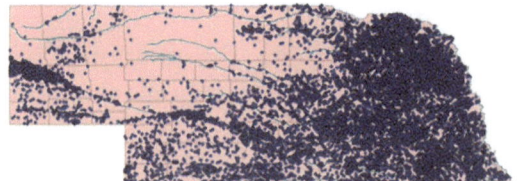

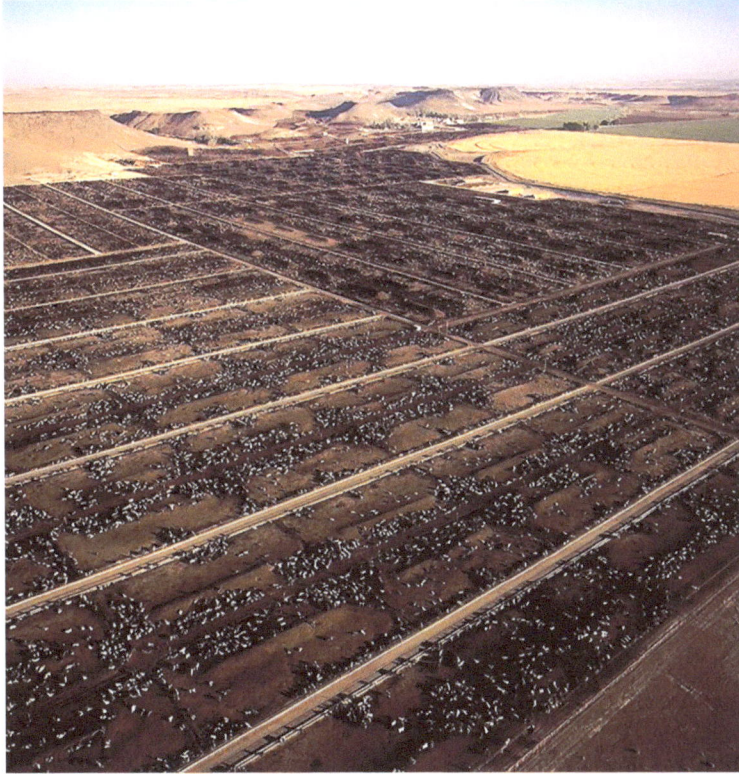

As far as the eye can see: Cattle whiling away the days stuffing themselves on grain and hay in Nebraska CAFOs.

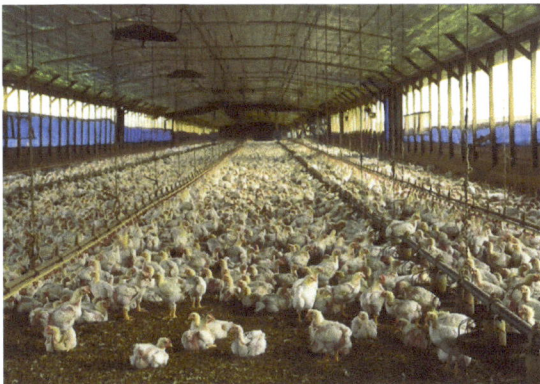

Marketing concept of "free-range" chickens, in which thousands of birds roam "cage free" in giant climate-controlled poultry houses. Commercially-raised chickens are fed grains exclusively.

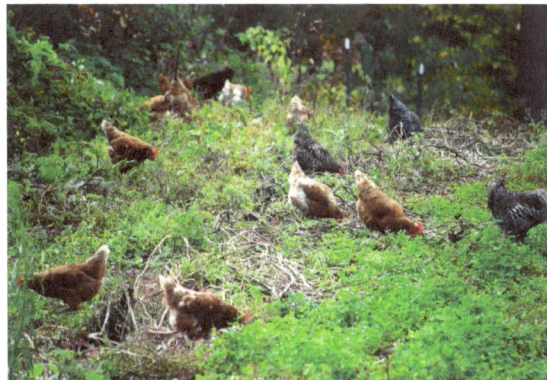

True free-range chickens, foraging for bugs, seeds, and green shoots. Chickens are natural omnivores and need a varied diet to thrive and produce nutritious eggs and meat.

Processed (Manufactured) Foods

Processed foods are little more than a base of refined carbohydrates such as white flour and sugar; HFCS (high-fructose corn syrup); refined, chemically extracted grain and seed oils; salt; and preservatives. These "pseudo-foods" have an unnaturally long shelf-life (sometimes years), as they are unappealing to and unable to support the life of bacteria, molds, insects, and rodents that might otherwise attempt to live off them.

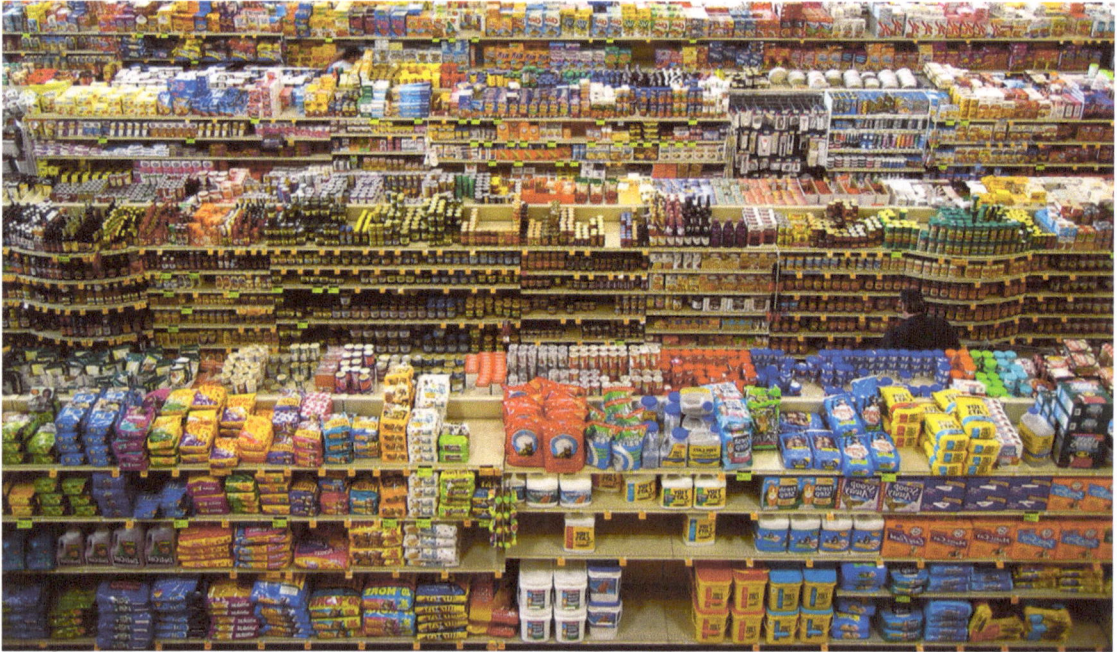

Row upon row of processed junk food occupies shelves in the modern grocery store. Our inflating wasitlines and the five diseases of modern society (metabolic syndrome, diabetes, arthritis, heart-disease, and cancer) are directly attribuable to consuming these processed food-stuffs over a life-time.

Processed foods are often referred to by nutritionists as "empty calories" or "anti-nutrients," because they do not provide significant vitamins, minerals, and enzymes required for their metabolism. These "food-like substances" instead *deplete* the body of vitamin, mineral, and enzyme stores, creating a nutritional deficit. For example, high sugar intake interferes with the body's assimilation of vitamin C (ascorbic acid is a *hexose,* a six-carbon sugar that behaves like a co-enzyme). Both refined sugar and vitamin C require the same enzymes and compete for the same transport pathways.

Most processed foods possess little to no fiber, and have been stripped of biologically active natural nutrients. Less active synthetic forms of nutrients are reintroduced by the food manufacturer to replace natural forms removed during processing. To add insult to injury, most processed foods contain high-fructose corn syrup (HFCS). HFCS is everywhere in processed foods—from sodas to candy bars to breakfast cereals, but much of it is "hidden" in products like salad dressing; condiments; frozen, boxed, or precooked dinners; bakery goods; dairy products; fast foods; snack foods; and other non-sweet products. HFCS raises blood fats (triglycerides) and contributes significantly to the current obesity epidemic.

Most importantly, processing foods increases their absorption rate, causing dramatic surges in blood sugar levels that eventually lead to disease, such as type-2 diabetes, atherosclerosis, and heart disease. There is a direct, undeniable link between insulin levels and disease, which will be discussed later in "Health Concepts #5—Dieting Strategies."

> Ancel Keys of the *The Seven Countries Study,* believed that dietary fat caused heart disease. We now know that there were actually 22 countries in the study, and 7 were "cherry-picked" to prove his Fat Hypothesis. Dr. Keys mistakenly assumed correlation is causation, a scientific mistake so fundamentally erroneous, it's rarely committed by a seasoned researcher, but more likely the blunder of a student. Worse, the study was done on sucrose/fat combination, villainizing the fat portion, but *ignoring the effect of the sugar!*

The self-appointed authoritarian organization, The American Heart Association, in 1961 began advancing the idea that fat (especially saturated) causes heart disease, with *zero* evidence or research to support it!

Processed foods are frequently loaded with fat (unless they are commercial "diet" foods that have had the fat replaced with sugar and HFCS to lower Calories), but not the healthy fats that promote health. Instead, manufacturers rely solely on the least expense fat sources available: chemically extracted and refined grain and seed oils. Soy, cotton, corn, safflower, and other seed (as opposed to nut or fruit) oils are extremely high in polyunsaturated fats. Once thought healthful for humans, new research indicates that diets high in polyunsaturates—in particular, a specific polyunsaturate called *arachidonic acid*—promote inflammatory processes leading to cancer, heart disease, joint disease, and type-2 diabetes. In addition to very high polyunsaturate levels, many processed foods often also contain hydrogenated fats. These fats have been artificially saturated to stabilize them, and are known to cause heart disease and other metabolic ills. The different fats will be discussed more thoroughly in the "Dietary Fats" section.

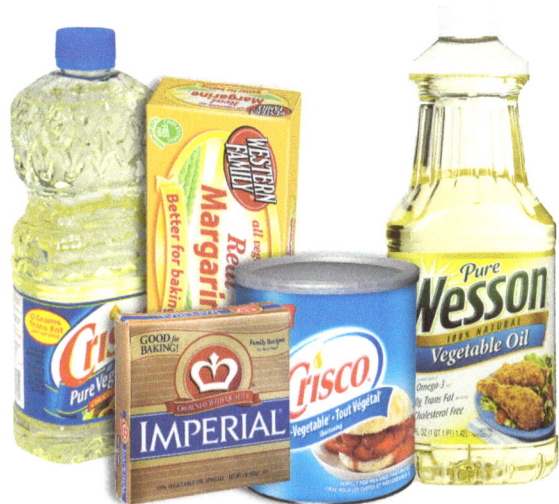

The Conspiracy to Keep Us Fat

Most of the consumer confusion with nutrition is a direct result of governmental policy vs. good science. The two paradigms are completely incompatible. The government's "Food Pyramid" and "My Plate" promote grains as the basis of a healthy diet with the majority of Calories coming from the "grain level," flying in the face of scientific evidence completely at odds with this nutritional protocol. While the First Lady lectures us on eating healthfully to control weight and prevent disease, her husband forks over yet another grain or sugar subsidy to keep the farmers growing the very substances that are responsible for our declining health and expanding waistlines. (Grains will be covered in more detail under Health Concept # 3.)

Fast food is everywhere you go—several establishments inhabit every block of typical urban areas. The populace is bombarded with images of fast food from television commercials, billboards, magazine and Internet advertisements, and radio announcements. It's almost impossible to avoid these images and the temptations that accompany them.

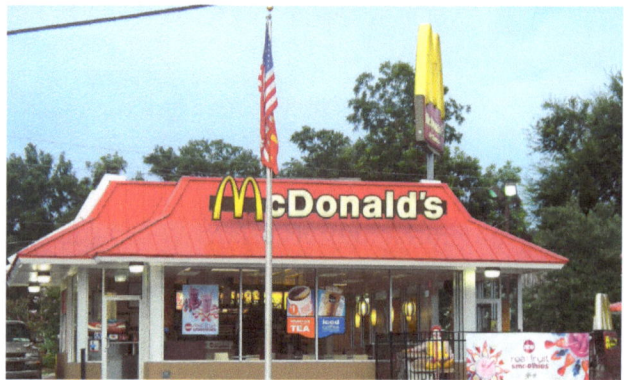

Many industries *profit* from obesity. Besides the processed food marketer's huge profits (a record $118 billion in sales for 2013), the diet industry is booming ($61 billion in profits for 2013); plus-size clothing sales are skyrocketing; large vehicles are selling better than ever; airlines can charge extra for larger passengers; all-you-can-eat buffets are packed; doctors, hospitals, and pharmaceutical companies profit from the continued rise in diabetes and its complications—amputations, blindness, kidney failure, and heart disease, in addition to joint surgeries and cancer treatments. Pharmaceutical companies rake it in for diabetes prescriptions and testing equipment while perpetually racing to release the newest miracle drug for controlling blood sugar. Obesity and hyperinsulinemia are very good indeed for revenue and the GNP.

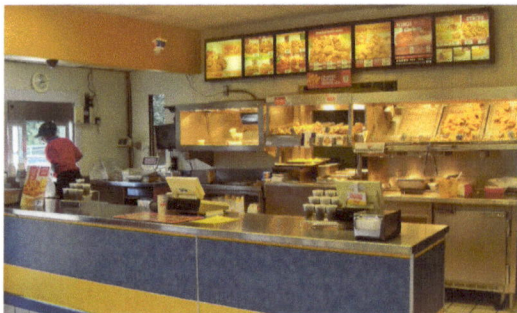

The United States Government is heavily involved in dietary recommendations, from a federal to a local level. Do you really believe that the government has any business telling you what to eat? Does it make sense that the government subsidizes grain and sugar crops, while restricting the size of soda the public may purchase? Is that *really* the government's purpose? Or is it *some other agenda*?

HEALTH CONCEPT #1

Your Body's Energy Balance

Energy is the ability to bring about change or to do work. Energy can be classified as either *potential* or *kinetic,* and exists in many forms: chemical, elastic, gravitational, magnetic, sound, electrical, light, mechanical, nuclear, and thermal.

Thermodynamics is the study of energy— the interrelation between heat (thermal energy), work, and the internal *potential energy* of a system. Thermodynamics is the domain of closed, non-living systems, such as stars in space and some atomic reactions.

Most people erroneously believe that the Laws of Thermodynamics pertain directly to life, and that:

Change in Mass = Energy In – Energy Out

This First Law of Thermodynamics (the conservation law) pertains *only to closed systems.* Living things are *not* closed systems.

The Second Law of Thermodynamics (also known as the Law of Entropy) is the measure of the disorder or randomness of energy and matter in a *closed system.* A closed system does not receive energy from outside the system, so the entropy increases, augmenting randomness within the system.

Because living beings are *not* closed systems, they require energy input from outside them to maintain life. Living matter is *ordered,* therefore it has low entropy. In biological systems, the Second Law of Thermodynamics governs how matter is converted to energy, and how some energy is converted back to matter again, as in gaining adipose tissue, building muscle, or forming a baby when pregnant. Entropy predominates only during disease and the aging process that leads to eventual death. However, the First and Second Laws of Thermodynamics are incomplete explanations for weight gain. Fat accumulation is a problem of *biology, not* physics! Body mass is regulated by hormones and enzymes, *not* how much we eat or how sedentary we are.

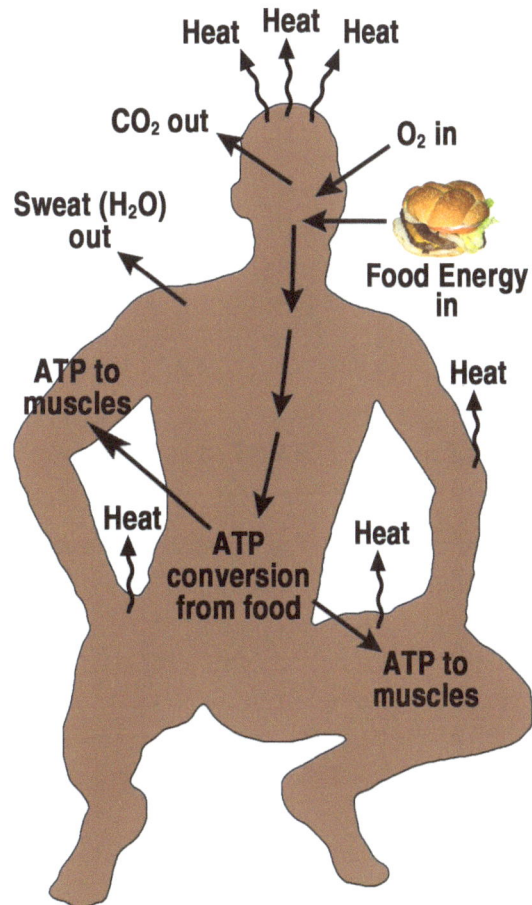

- Food contains Potential Energy. Potential energy is energy that has not yet been used.

- When food is burned (in the presence of oxygen—that's why we need to breathe it), Potential Energy converts to Kinetic Energy—energy in use (or motion). Some of the kinetic energy is transformed to chemical energy in our bodies; the rest is lost as thermal energy (heat). The chemical energy is measured in kilo-calories, or Calories for short. The heat generated by burning dietary Calories is what generates our body temperature.

Energy Input

Food biochemical energy contains potential energy and kinetic energy. One pound of sugar has a certain potential energy. If that pound of sugar is burned, the energy is released as kinetic energy (chemical reactions and heat). So much heat is released, in fact, that organisms would combust if all the energy were released at once. Organisms must release the energy a little bit at a time. *Enzymes* and *hormones* regulate the *rate* at which energy converts and is released and transformed from potential to kinetic forms.

Energy balance depends largely on how your hormones and enzymes help you burn food, store and release fat, and how your body responds to exercise. It is simply *not true* that weight stabilizes when calories in equals calories burned. This is way too simplistic of a picture for such a complex process! We all know someone thin who eats like a ravenous hyena on the Serengeti day after day, but gains no weight. We may know—or even be— one of the unfortunate souls who maintains the same weight on few calories, eating very little. *Let's read that again:*

Change in Mass Does *NOT* = Calories In – Calories Burned

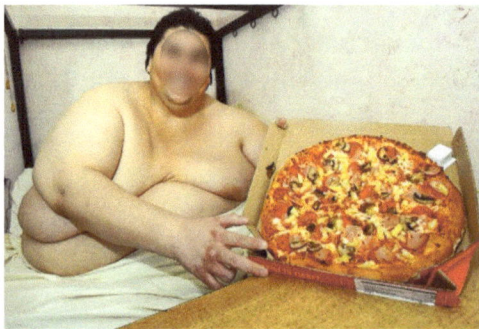

Obesity is a matter of fat accumulation, *not* increased energy *in* (gluttony), or reduced energy *out* (sloth). Overeating and inactivity are *compensatory* mechanisms; they are *not causes*. We don't get fat because we overeat; we overeat because our fat tissue is accumulating excess fat, leaving less energy for bodily processes *other* than fat accumulation. Important cells are starving and are literally malnourished while the fat compiles. Fat accumulation creates relentless hunger, and that hunger drives overeating. So, the logical question is then, "What is causing fat to accumulate?" The answer is *hormones*.

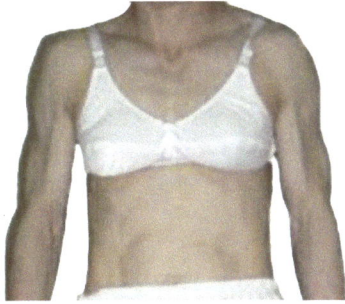

Is this person overweight?

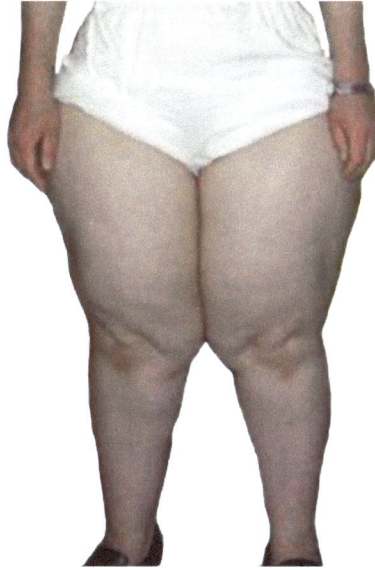

Is *THIS* person overweight?

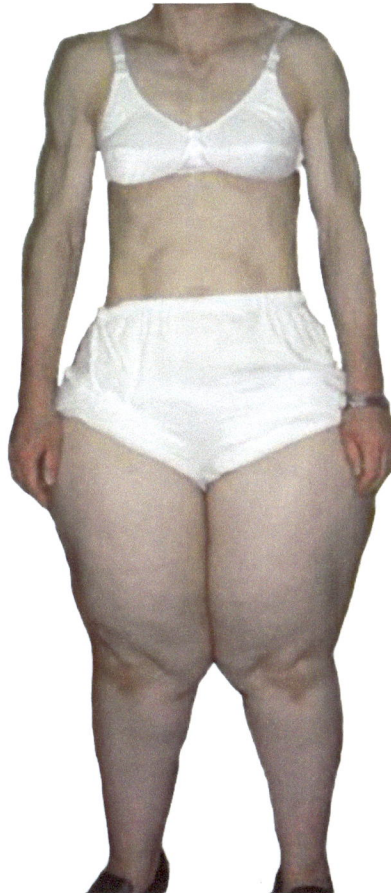

How about *THIS* person—is she overweight?

Do you think this person ate boxes of donuts—*willful* donuts that decided to go to the lower half of her body, ignoring the top half? This does not—*cannot*—happen! These distorted fat accumulations are due to a condition called *lipodystrophy* (meaning "fat disorder")—governed strictly by *hormones.* This bizarre redistribution of fat, in which fat loss occurs above the waist while it accumulates below the waist, occurs mostly in women. Females comprise 80% of lipodystrophy cases. Though lipodystrophy is an extreme example of hormone imbalance, the same mechanisms govern fat accumulation in average people.

The rate at which energy is burned (output) varies considerably from person to person because of the unique makeup of their *hormone and enzyme profiles.* These components primarily regulate weight gain or loss. Many factors influence your hormone and enzyme profile, but your profile *can* change with diet and (surprisingly little) exercise. More on hormones and enzymes later.

In 1929, Gustav von Bergmaan and Julius Bauer proposed the Lipophilia Hypothesis, in which certain cells seize energy from foodstuffs and store it, even in nutritionally-deprived states. Genetically-engineered "Zucker" rats get fatter when they eat less—even the brain and other organs are cannibalized to store more fat. Lipogenesis increases independently of the nutritional requirements of the organism, acting as almost a *separate organ* or tumor. Fat accumulates even in subjects half-starved!

Your hormones and enzymes can be fine tuned, so you run like a Ferrari rather than an overloaded Hoopty. Have you ever thought of your body as a biological internal combustion engine? *It actually is!*

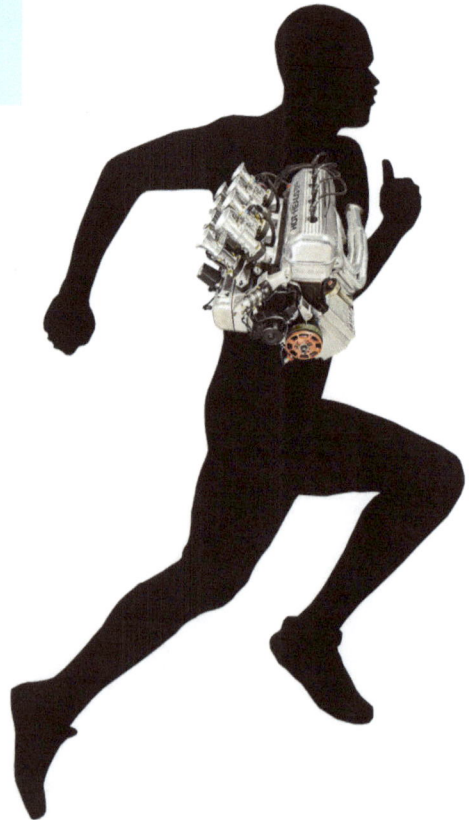

Energy Output

What Governs Biological Energy Transformations?

The transformation of food into energy for your body is called *metabolism.* Metabolic processes are primarily mediated through enzymes and hormones. Hormones especially, determine the differences between individuals and their energy levels and weight equilibrium. These hormones, in turn, are directly influenced by diet and activity levels, and to a lesser—but significant extent—by genetics, illness, and pharmaceuticals.

We will discuss two factors—diet and exercise—in this book, because they are the two constituents you can directly do something about. The other three determinants of weight and metabolism—genetics, illness, and pharmaceuticals—may or may not be under your control, depending on your circumstances.

Your individual genetics provide a template—a *potential*—of how your body will tend to use and burn energy, and store and burn fat, because your hormone and enzyme profile is partially inherited. Energy levels and weight run in families, however, genetics isn't an intractable fixed factor that cannot be influenced. Environmental factors such as diet and exercise can alter the *expression* of genes you inherited (called *epigenetics*)—genes can be turned on and off with proper encouragement.

Illness—either acute or chronic—can affect weight management. Being bedridden or wheelchair-bound can cause fat gain combined with muscle and bone loss. Inactivity—especially of the legs, which act like a second heart—is deleterious to your health. Inactivity weakens the heart and accelerates aging and disease processes, leading to blood sugar problems and fat accumulation while muscles atrophy. Chronic diseases such as emphysema and tuberculosis can cause weight *loss*—especially of muscle tissue, due to oxygen deprivation that prevents food from being burned efficiently, among other processes, the discussion of which is beyond the scope of this book.

Prescription drugs can make you fat by altering enzymes and hormones. Drug-induced diabetes can occur most notably from prolonged use of *glucocorticoids*—corticosteroids used for intractable pain or autoimmune disease. Drug-induced hyperglycemia or diabetes may also occur with prolonged treatment with several other drug classes as listed in the table on the next page.

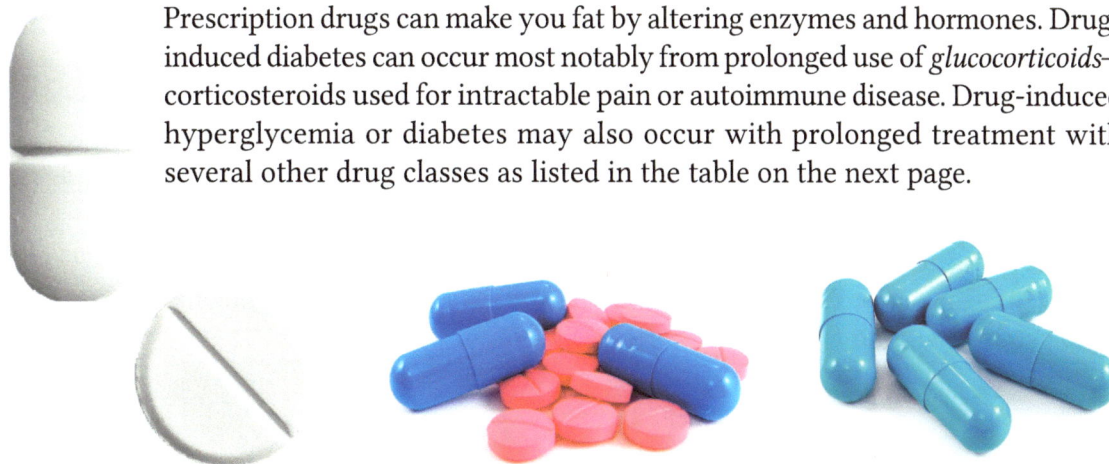

Drugs that Cause Hyperglycemia or Diabetes	
DRUG	PRESCRIBED FOR
Albuterol (inhaler)	asthma (acute)
Amphotericin B	fungal infections
Atorvastatin (Lipitor®)	high cholesterol
Baclofen	muscle relaxant and peripheral nerve damage, especially spinal nerve roots
Beta-blockers (Metoprolol, Atenolol, Carvedilol, Nadolol, etc.)	hypertension and heart arrhythmias
Caffeine (large amounts)	stimulant
Captopril (ACE inhibitor)	hypertension
Cyclosporine	psoriasis, immunosuppressant (anti-rejection in organ transplants)
Estradiol, Levonorgestrel, Medroxyprogesterone, Norgestrel (synthetic female hormones)	birth control, menopause, irregular menstruation
Furosemide (Lasix®)	diuretic for hypertension or congestive heart failure (CHF)
Glucocorticoids (a class of Corticosteroids)	debilitating pain and auto-immune disease
Glucosamine (intravenous)	joint damage or dysfunction
Interferon	anti-viral, immune booster
NSAIDs—Non-Steroidal Anti-Inflammatory Drugs (Indomethacin, diclofenac, etc.)	arthritis and joint, tendon, & ligament disorders
Phenytoin (Dilantin®)	epilepsy, spasms
Protease (an enzyme) inhibitors	anti-viral used for HIV/AIDS and hepatitis C; possible cancer treatment
Risperidone (Risperdal®)	psychosis, bipolar disorder (manic-depressive syndrome), schizophrenia, Tourette's syndrome
SSRIs—Selective Serotonin Re-uptake Inhibitors (Paxil®— paroxetine, Prozac®—fluoxetine)	clinical depression
Therapeutic doses of Niacin (>2,000 mgs./day)	high cholesterol

The above list is far from complete; consult a prescription drug reference, or an online resource such as HTTP://WWW.RxLIST.COM for more information.

Some of the hormones that regulate metabolism and fat storage are listed in the table on the next page. Note that fat cells secrete many hormones that regulate not only how fat is stored and released to be burned for energy, but influence other hormones. Adipose tissue (body fat) behaves more like an *organ*—producing its own hormones and enzymes—rather than act as just storage for extra calories!

Hormones and Enzymes that Regulate Metabolism and Fat Storage		
HORMONE	**SECRETED FROM**	**ACTIVITY**
Insulin	pancreas	transports sugar from the blood to inside cells; accelerates fat storage and blocks leptin signaling so fat doesn't break down for energy
Glucagon	liver	breaks down stored glycogen for sugar
Human Growth Hormone (HGH or Somatotropin)	pituitary	increases lay-down of lean muscle tissue; accelerates fat breakdown
Thyroxine	thyroid	regulates rate of energy conversion
Cortisol	adrenal glands	stimulates release of epinephrine, which causes break down of glycogen from muscle and liver; increases blood sugar
Epinephrine	adrenal glands	helps release glycogen from liver and muscles
Leptin	fat cells	stimulates stored fat (adipose) breakdown for energy
Adiponectin	fat cells	increases cellular sensitivity to insulin; regulates fat storage
Tumor necrosis factor-α (TNF-α)	fat cells	increases inflammation, leads to cancerous tumor growth
Resistin	fat cells	increases insulin resistance, leading to type-2 diabetes
IL-6 (interleukin-6)	immune and fat cells	increases insulin resistance; leads to high blood fats (hyperlipidemia); may also reduce adiponectin secretion
Ghrelin	stomach lining	increases appetite and cravings, especially in high-insulin states; low to moderate exercise reduces grehlin secretion, thereby reducing appetite
Cholecystokinin (CCK)	small intestine	suppresses appetite in presence of fats; low-fat diets inhibit its release, increasing hunger
Lipoprotein lipase	enzyme in fat cells and muscle tissue	inhibits fat storage, accelerates lipolysis (breakdown of fat for energy)
TPPII (Tripeptidyl peptidase II	intracellular enzyme	promotes fat formation, increases hunger

Investigation of these 15 hormones and enzymes and how they interrelate is beyond the scope of this book, but interested readers may find more information in nutritional biochemistry books and on the Internet. *Nutritional Self-Defense: Better Health in a Polluted, Over-Processed, and Stressful World* by the author, is a more in-depth excursion into metabolic biochemistry. A great Internet source is the *Journal of Clinical Endocrinology & Metabolism,* at: HTTP://JCEM.ENDOJOURNALS.ORG/

HEALTH CONCEPT #2

Calories from Macro-Nutrients

Health experts generally agree that there is macro-nutrient *ratio* that leads to good health, in which there is an optimal balance of the three macro-nutrients: carbohydrates, proteins, and fats. The generally accepted ratios of carbohydrate are 50–60%, protein 15–20%, and fats 25–30%, appearing in the table below for two typical Calorie levels. In general, women require fewer Calories than men because they possess less metabolizing muscle tissue, and therefore have a somewhat slower metabolism. These ratios may need to be altered for people with special considerations. Those who are professional athletes, are obese, wheelchair-bound, recovering from injury, or have other medical issues will require a modified diet plan recommended by a qualified health professional with expertise in nutrition.

Calories per Gram of Nutrient: Carbohydrate = **4** Protein = **4** Fat = **9** Alcohol = **7**

	1200 CALORIES (WEIGHT REDUCTION)			**2000 CALORIES (AVERAGE INTAKE)**		
Macro-Nutrient Ratio of "Ideal" Diets						
PARAMETER	C	P	F	C	P	**F**
Calories	600	240	360	1200	300	500
Grams	150	60	40	300	75	56
Percentage	50%	20%	30%	60%	15%	25%

Percentages of macro-nutrients are calculated in the following manner:

(Macro-Nutrient Calories/Total Calories) x 100 = Caloric Percentage
(Example: (600/1200) = 0.50 x 100 = 50%)

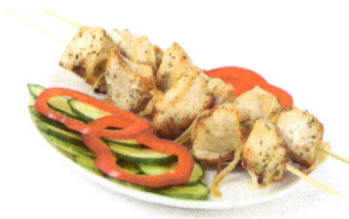

Instructions

Fill out the Food Journal on the next page using the Food Composition tables found at the back this book. You will continually refer to your Food Journal to do the calculations in many of the Self-Assessment activities, so bookmark this page.

Your 24-Hour Food Journal						
FOOD	AMOUNT	CALORIES	C	P	F	FIBER
BREAKFAST						
LUNCH						
DINNER						
DESSERT						
SNACKS & BEVERAGES						
		CALORIES	C	P	F	FI

Self-Assessment

Enter the total Calories consumed in a day: _____

1. Enter the *total grams* of each of the macro-nutrients:

    Carbohydrates: _____ Proteins: _____ Fats: _____

2. Enter the *percentages* of carbohydrates, proteins, and fats in your diet.

    Macro-Nutrient Calories/Total Calories) x 100 = Caloric Percentage

    Carbohydrates: _____ Proteins: _____ Fats: _____

3. How close are your percentages to the chart on page 24?

4. Is there room for improvement?

5. What might you adjust to improve your nutritional health?

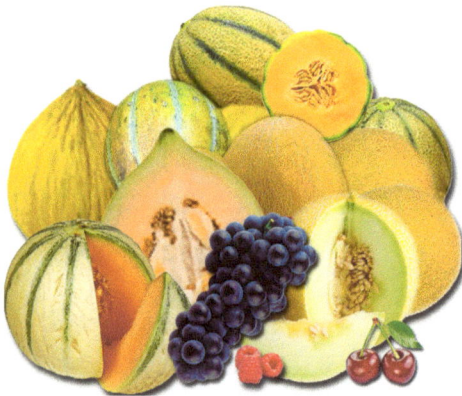

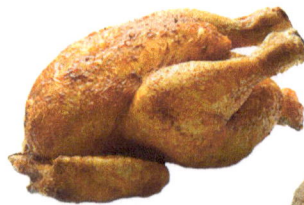

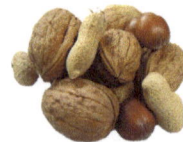

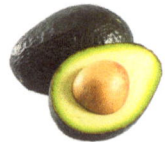

HEALTH CONCEPT #3

Macro-Nutrients in Food

Macro-nutrients include carbohydrates (sugars and starches), protein (both animal and plant sources), and fats (from both animal and plant sources). Ideal human diets contain all of the macro-nutrients in balance with each other, as imbalances cause disease. See the following table for a quick rundown on what happens when too little or too much of a macro-nutrient is present in the diet for prolonged periods:

Macro-Nutrients: Effects of Quantity Distortion		
MACRO-NUTRIENT	**TOO LITTLE**	**TOO MUCH**
Carbohydrates (sugars and starches)	causes *ketosis*, a state in which fat is preferentially burned for fuel. Can stress or damage the kidneys and lead to a starvation state and pronounced muscle loss if not balanced with increased protein and fat.	causes weight gain, hyperglycemia (increased blood sugar), which leads to diabetes. Also results in high blood triglycerides and cholesterol imbalance with increased LDLs and decreased HDLs.
Protein (mostly animal source)	causes muscle tissue wasting, a swollen liver (leading to *marasmus* or *kwashiorkor*), and serious enzyme, hormone, and neurotransmitter under-production	damages the kidneys, causes dehydration and mineral loss that may result in serious disease states, and may cause cancer
Lipids (fats)	causes reduced hormone production, malabsorption of fat-soluble vitamins and minerals, and increased hunger	causes cancer and other inflammatory disease states (especially from the processed polyunsaturate type). It is the *kind of fat* in the diet, rather than the quantity of fat, that is of vital concern for health.

Carbohydrates

Carbohydrates are the body's immediate energy source and are "protein-sparing," in that they prevent muscle tissue breakdown for immediate fuel. For healthy and active individuals, carbohydrates are vitally important to well-being. Individual requirements may vary greatly from 20–1000 grams daily, depending on age, metabolic rate, activity level, blood sugar levels, and ratio to other macro-nutrients (protein and fats).

Carbohydrates should generally comprise 50–60% of a healthful diet for a generally healthy individual. The majority of these carbohydrates should derive from plants such as fresh vegetables and fruits. New research indicates that whole grains—though an acceptable part of most diets—are best consumed in far lesser quantities than originally thought to be conducive to good health. Current research in glycemic response confirms that complex carbohydrates are not necessarily more slowly absorbed than simpler carbohydrates. High-glycemic foods (carbohydrates that cause a dramatic rise in blood sugar) stimulate your body to produce excess insulin and arachidonic acid, which causes inflammation. Diets very high in grains—even whole grains, but especially refined grain products—lead to disease states. Over-consumption of grain products causes obesity. The marbling prized in a gourmet beef steak is a direct result of grain. If you need to gain weight, load up on grain products!

Carbohydrates take 2–5 hours to digest. Fats are digested slowly over a 5–8 hour period. Fats retard carbohydrate absorption by slowing stomach emptying. In small amounts, fat can be beneficial in this respect, as in adding a small amount of butter or sour cream to a baked potato (a quickly-absorbed food when plain—see *"Glycemic Index and Glycemic Load"* on page 86 under "Health Concept #5—Dieting Strategies"). Moderation and *balance* are the secrets to feeling good!

Carbohydrate (Saccharide) Classes		
SIMPLE	COMPOUND (COMPLEX)	# MOLECULES
Monosaccharides		1 saccharide
Disaccharides		2 monosaccharides
Trisaccharides		3 monosaccharides
Oligosaccharides		a chain of up to 10 monosaccharides
	Polysaccharides (starches and glycogen)	hundreds to thousands of oligosaccharides chained together

An easy way to recognize a sugar is by its name: Words ending in "ose" usually indicate some kind of sugar. You may discover many kinds of sugars disguised in food labels—sucr*ose*, fruct*ose*, gluc*ose*, dextr*ose*, levul*ose*, galact*ose*, etc. Just look for the "ose" in the labels, and you've found the sugar. All carbohydrates eventually break down to glucose.

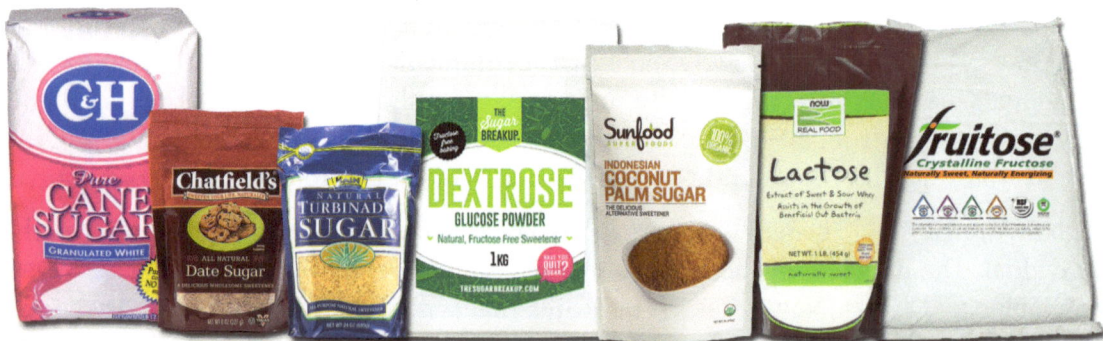

The Saccharides (sugars & starches)

I.   MONOSACCHARIDES
   A.   **Tetroses** ($C_4H_8O_4$)
      1)   Erythrose
   B.   **Pentoses** ($C_5H_{10}O_5$)
      1)   Arabinose
      2)   Xylose
      3)   Ribose
      4)   Lyxose
   C.   **Hexoses** ($C_6H_{12}O_6$)
      1)   Aldohexoses

         a)   glucose (a.k.a. dextrose)...(zymase $\rightarrow$ ethanol + CO_2)
         b)   galactose
         c)   mannose
         d)   gulose
         e)   idose
         f)   talose
         g)   altrose
         h)   allose
      2)   Ketohexoses
         a)   fructose (levulose)
         b)   sorbose
         c)   tagatose

II.   DISACCHARIDES ($C_{12}H_{22}O_{11}$)
   A.   **Sucrose**...(invertase $\rightarrow$ glucose + fructose)
   B.   **Lactose**...(lactase $\rightarrow$ glucose + galactose)
   C.   **Maltose**...(maltase $\rightarrow$ 2 glucose)
   D.   **Melibiose**...(enzymes or dilute acid $\rightarrow$ glucose + galactose)
   E.   **Cellobiose**...(maltase or cellase $\rightarrow$ 2 glucose)
   F.   **Trehalose**

III.   TRISACCHARIDES ($C_{18}H_{32}O_{16}$)
   A.   **Raffinose** (melitose)...(invertase $\rightarrow$ fructose + melibiose; emulsin $\rightarrow$ sucrose + galactose)

IV.   POLYSACCHARIDES ($C_6H_{10}O_5$)
   A.   **Starches**...(diastase $\rightarrow$ maltose; maltase or acids $\rightarrow$ glucose)
   B.   **Cellulose**...(HCl + heat $\rightarrow$ glucose; acetic anhydride + concentrated sulfuric acid $\rightarrow$ cellobiose)
   C.   **Dextrin**...(diastase $\rightarrow$ maltose; maltase or acids $\rightarrow$ glucose)
   D.   **Inulin**...(inulase $\rightarrow$ fructose)
   E.   **Glycogen**...(diastase or ptyalin $\rightarrow$ glucose + maltose)
   F.   **Pentosans**

You may remember from high-school biology that the basic energy molecule in living tissue is ATP (adenosine triphosphate). ATP is obtained from metabolizing *glucose* through several transitions with the help of enzymes, mediated by vitamins and minerals.

Glycolysis (simplified)

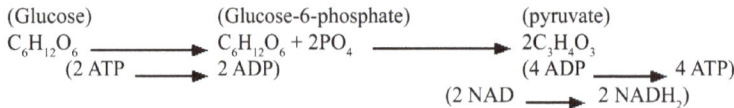

(Glucose) → (Glucose-6-phosphate) → (pyruvate) | **First Stage Glycolysis**

$$C_6H_{12}O_6 \longrightarrow C_6H_{12}O_6 + 2PO_4 \longrightarrow 2C_3H_4O_3$$
$$(2\ ATP \longrightarrow 2\ ADP) \qquad (4\ ADP \longrightarrow 4\ ATP)$$
$$(2\ NAD \longrightarrow 2\ NADH_2)$$

Anaerobic Respiration

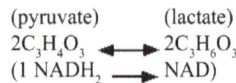

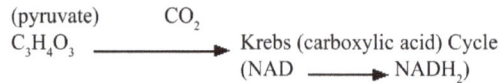

Accounting:

(pyruvate) (lactate)
$$2C_3H_4O_3 \longleftarrow 2C_3H_6O_3$$
$$(1\ NADH_2 \longrightarrow NAD)$$

Accounting:

2 pyruvates
2 $NADH_2$
2 ATP

4 $NADH_2$ (x2)
1 $FADH_2$ (x2)
1 ATP (x2)

Aerobic Respiration

(pyruvate) CO_2
$$C_3H_4O_3 \longrightarrow \text{Krebs (carboxylic acid) Cycle}$$
$$(NAD \longrightarrow NADH_2)$$

Citric Acid Cycle

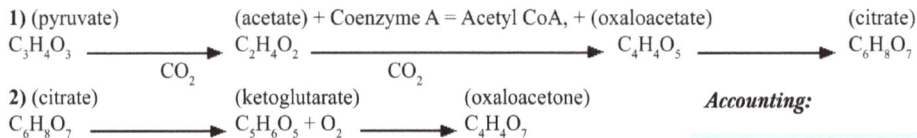

1) (pyruvate) (acetate) + Coenzyme A = Acetyl CoA, + (oxaloacetate) (citrate)
$$C_3H_4O_3 \longrightarrow C_2H_4O_2 \longrightarrow C_4H_4O_5 \longrightarrow C_6H_8O_7$$
$$\qquad CO_2 \qquad\qquad CO_2$$

2) (citrate) (ketoglutarate) (oxaloacetone)
$$C_6H_8O_7 \longrightarrow C_5H_6O_5 + O_2 \longrightarrow C_4H_4O_7$$

Accounting:

2 NAD $\longrightarrow$ $NADH_2$
1 ADP $\longrightarrow$ ATP
1 FAD $\longrightarrow$ $FADH_2$

Electron Transport System

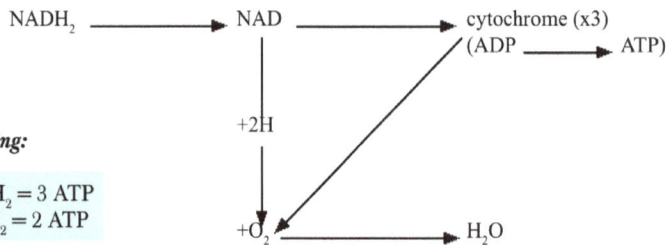

$$NADH_2 \longrightarrow NAD \longrightarrow \text{cytochrome (x3)}$$
$$(ADP \longrightarrow ATP)$$
$$+2H$$
$$+O_2 \longrightarrow H_2O$$

Accounting:

1 $NADH_2$ = 3 ATP
1 $FADH_2$ = 2 ATP

LEGEND

AMP	adenosine monophosphate
ADP	adenosine diphosphate
ATP	adenosine triphosphate
NAD	nicotinamide adenine dinucleotide
NADH₂	nicotinamide adenine dinucleotide + 2 e⁻ in H bonds
NADPH	nicotinamide adenine dinucleotide + PO_4 and 1 H bond
FAD	flavin adenine dinucleotide
FADH₂	flavin adenine dinucleotide + 2H (e⁻)

Total:

38 ATP
3 electron transport

Fiber: The Indigestible Carbohydrate

Dietary fiber is essential for good health. Fiber does not provide energy Calories for humans, as humans lack the digestive enzymes necessary to break fiber down and derive nutrition from it (unlike most herbivores like cattle, horses, goats, etc.). Health professionals recommend consuming at least 14 grams of fiber daily for every 1000 Calories consumed, up to 25–40 grams. Generally, fiber intake will be adequate when the bulk of the diet consists of vegetables, fruits, and legumes, with modest amounts of whole grains. Processed foods are generally devoid of fiber unless it has been added as a marketing strategy for increasing profits.

Dietary fiber comes in two varieties: soluble and insoluble. Soluble fiber (as found in beans, peas, lentils, oats, nuts, seeds, psyllium, apples, pears, strawberries, and blueberries) slows the absorption of carbohydrates by increasing the number of glucose receptor sites in the intestine, assisting in blood sugar regulation, which helps prevent type-2 diabetes. Soluble fiber lowers LDL (bad) cholesterol, reducing the risk of heart disease.

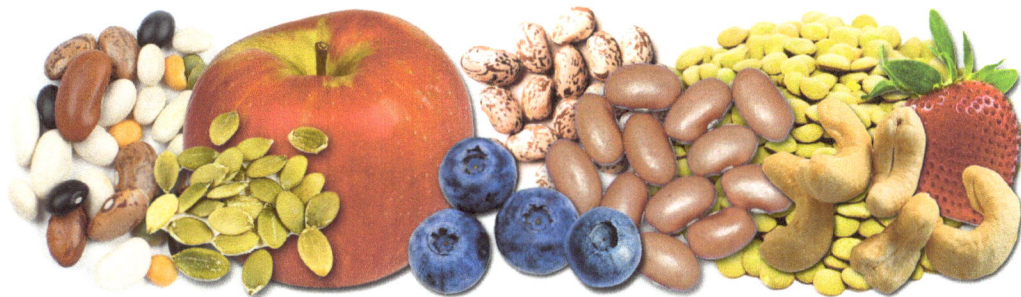

Legumes, fruits, nuts, and seeds are high in soluble fiber.

Insoluble fiber—as found in whole grains such as barley, brown rice, wheat bran; and nuts, seeds, carrots, cucumbers, zucchini, celery, green beans, dark leafy vegetables—encourages favorable bacterial growth, which aids in the digestion of starches and serves as "nature's broom" to assist in elimination. The bacterial cultures that thrive in fiber-rich environments manufacture B-vitamins such as biotin and niacin, essential to health. An added benefit is that fiber reduces hunger.

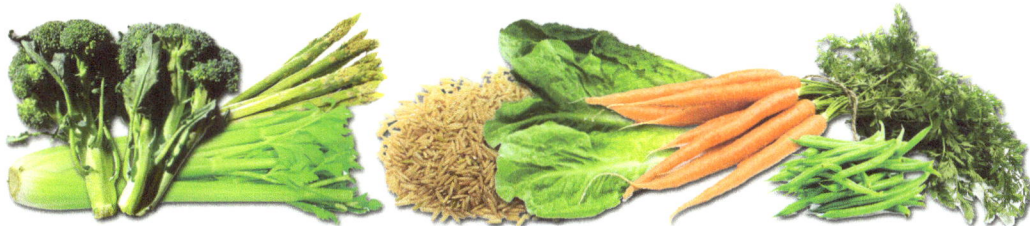

Insoluble fiber as found in grains and most fibrous vegetables, are essential to intestinal health.

One of the most important features of fiber is its fat-sequestering activity. Fiber traps some of the fat molecules in the colon, allowing them to move undigested out of the body. In fact, the higher the saturated fat content of your diet, the higher the fiber content should be to ensure that fat molecules quickly move out of the body rather than staying in the colon forming potentially carcinogenic metabolites.

Compounds Produced when Fiber Intake is Inadequate		
COMPOUND	SOURCE	DISEASE STATE
Alcohol (Ethanol)	alcoholic beverages	cancers throughout digestive system and breast
Azoxymethane	grain-fed beef fat	colon cancer
Lithocholate	dietary saturated fat	causes the liver to reduce the conversion of cholesterol into bile salts, increasing serum cholesterol
Apocholic acid	bacterial putrefaction and breakdown of bile acids	colon cancer
3-methyl-cholanthrene	bacterial putrefaction and breakdown of bile acids	colon cancer
Nitrosamines	nitrates from both natural plants (commercially-grown with chemical fertilizers) and processed (cured) meats, such as bacon and lunch meats	colon cancer
Fecapentanes	bacterial putrefaction and breakdown of bile acids	colon cancer

It is possible to overindulge in fiber. Fiber—especially grain fiber—contains *phytic acid* (phytate) that binds to minerals. Excess fiber in the diet can therefore hinder the absorption of calcium, magnesium, zinc, and other minerals, creating serious nutritional deficiencies.

Instructions

Use the Fiber Table on the next three pages to help you fill out your Food Journal.

Fiber Table		
FOOD	**AMOUNT**	**GRAMS**
Apple, raw	1 medium	5.40
Apricots, dried	1 cup	11.70
Artichoke	1 medium	7.20
Asparagus	1 cup	2.85
Avocado	½ medium	1.80
Barley, dry	1 cup	2.10
Beans, Garbanzo, cooked	1 cup	10.00
Beans, green, cooked	1 cup	3.60
Beans, kidney, cooked	1 cup	8.34
Beans, lima, cooked	1 cup	9.00
Beans, pinto, cooked	1 cup	7.20
Blackberries, raw	1 cup	17.70
Boysenberries, raw	1 cup	10.14
Bran, rice	1 cup	7.20
Bran, wheat	1 cup	10.40
Bread, hotdog bun	1	0
Bread, pumpernickel	1 slice	1.20
Bread, white enriched	1 slice	0
Bread, whole wheat	1 slice	1.20
Broccoli, cooked	1 cup	6.00
Brussels sprouts, cooked	1 cup	6.30
Cabbage, raw	1 cup	2.40
Cantaloupe	½ medium	1.80
Carrots, raw	1 large	3.00
Celery, raw	1 cup	2.10
Cherries, sweet, raw	1 cup	1.56
Coconut meat	1 cup	8.10
Corn meal	1 cup	3.60
Corn, canned	1 cup	3.30
Crackers, graham	1 large	.66
Crackers, RyKrisp	2	.90
Cucumber	1 cup	1.80
Dates, pitted	10	6.90
Figs, dried	2	3.60
Grapes	1 cup	2.40
Guava, raw	1 medium	16.80
Hominy, cooked	1 cup	.60

Fiber Table, continued		
FOOD	AMOUNT	GRAMS
Kumquat	1	2.22
Lentils, cooked	1 cup	7.20
Lettuce, iceberg	1 cup	1.05
Macaroni, enriched, cooked	1 cup	.30
Mango, raw	1 medium	8.10
Millet, dry	1 cup	21.90
Muffin, bran	1	2.16
Muffin, English	1	0
Mushrooms, cooked	1 cup	0
Noodles, egg, cooked	1 cup	.60
Nuts, almonds	2 oz	3.00
Nuts, Brazil	2 oz	4.10
Nuts, cashews, roasted	2 oz	1.50
Nuts, peanuts, roasted	2 oz	3.00
Oatmeal, cooked	1 cup	1.50
Orange	1 medium	2.70
Pancake	1—4" diameter	.30
Papaya	½ medium	5.40
Peach	1 medium	2.07
Pear	1 medium	8.40
Peas, canned	1 cup	11.70
Peppers, green bell	1 cup	3.36
Popcorn	1 cup	.90
Potato, russet, baked	1 medium	3.60
Prunes, dry	1 cup	6.60
Pumpkin seeds	2 oz	2.00
Pumpkin, canned	1 cup	3.60
Raspberries, raw	1 cup	12.00
Rice, brown, cooked	1 cup	1.35
Rice, white, cooked	1 cup	.60
Sauerkraut, canned	1 cup	6.00
Spinach, canned	1 cup	4.80
Spinach, raw	1 cup	.90
Squash, summer, cooked	1 cup	2.40
Squash, winter, cooked	1 cup	7.80
Sunflower seeds	2 oz	4.10
Tomato, raw	1 medium	2.40

Fiber Table, continued		
FOOD	AMOUNT	GRAMS
Tortilla, corn	1—6"	.90
Watermelon	6" x 1½"	5.40
Wheat, shredded	1 biscuit	1.50
Yams, cooked	1 cup	5.40

Self-Assessment

The National Cancer Institute, most dietitians, and nutritionists recommend a daily fiber (both soluble and insoluble) intake of 30–45 grams. Does your intake measure up, or is there room for improvement?

Modern Grains: The Staff of Life...?

Grains are the current hot controversy in nutritional circles. Many paleo-anthropologists and geneticists assert that grains are not necessarily an ideal food for humans—or even livestock, for that matter. Genetic change (adaptation) is excruciatingly slow. For example, it takes 500,000 years for 1% of mitochondrial DNA (the genetic material inherited only from our mothers) to mutate, and effect genetic change. It is quite possible we have not been eating grains long enough to have adapted to them. Conversely, Gregory Cochran and Henry Harpending, authors of *The 10,000 Year Explosion,* argue that humans have indeed adapted quite well to grains in just ten millennia, as grains are predominantly responsible for civilization accelerating human evolution.

History of Grains

Anthropologists and paleontologists have determined that for nearly two million years, the bulk of the *hominid* (human-like ancestors) diet consisted of mammals (including organs, fat, and bone marrow), cooked tubers (starchy and fibrous roots), seafood (including seaweed and tide-pool shellfish), nuts, berries, fruits, leaves and stems (green vegetation), fungi (mushrooms), birds, eggs, and insects. Humankind has been grain-free for most of its existence.

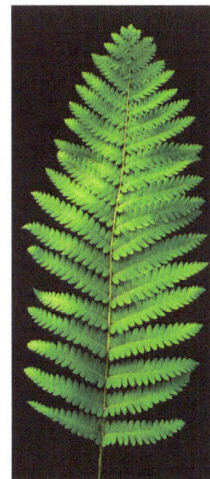

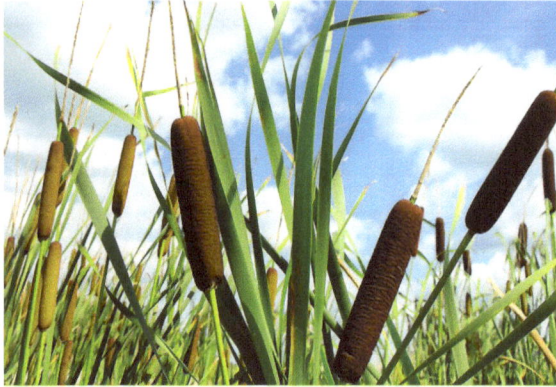

An article printed in *The Daily Mail* in October of 2010 declared that Stone-Age man had been eating bread for 30,000 years—way longer than previously thought. This revelation shook up researchers. The claim was later exposed as a case of bad journalism with a misleading conclusion. The devil is in the details: Humans 30,000 years ago did not eat grain-based bread; the substances they used to make a flour-like paste came from cattails and ferns—a far cry from any grain.

The first evidence of nutritionally significant grain crops (*emmer* and *einkorn*—ancestors of modern wheat) first appeared in the Fertile Crescent about 11,500 years ago. China began rice cultivation about 10,000 years ago, and the outset of corn domestication began in South America about 9,000 years ago. Paleo-anthropologists maintain that averaged over civilizations, humans have been eating significant quantities of grain-stuffs for about 10,000 years. More scrutiny reveals that Western Europe, such as the British Isles, weren't cultivating grains until 7,500 years ago, and corn dependency was not evident in the Americas until 1,200 years ago. North Americans adopted a grain-based diet less than 150 years ago.

Anthropologists can trace the adoption of grain-based diets to the decline of dental health in human fossils. Our modern health woes may be attributed to a surge of grain-product consumption (in addition to processed polyunsaturated oils and high-fructose corn syrup) that began in the 1940s, and the dramatic genetic modifications of modern wheat beginning in the 1960s.

The big attraction to grains is simply that grains can be stored for long periods, assuring against starvation during food scarcity. With grain in stock, large populations of humans can survive under a single ruler or religious ideology. Consequently, grain-based civilizations can conquer and expand into areas previously inhabited by hunter-gatherers. Cultivation, storing, processing, and trade in grains—specifically, ancient wheat relatives—marked the beginnings of civilization.

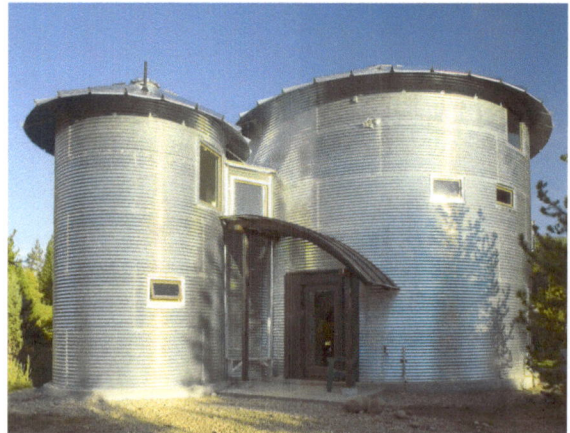

Modern Wheat

Modern wheat differs strikingly from ancient emmer and einkorn. Emmer has 14 chromosomes and einkorn has 28; modern wheat sports 42 chromosomes—almost as many as a human being (46). Ancient grain grasses grow up to six feet, but modern wheat is only two or three feet tall. Hybridization through selective breeding and gene modification have enhanced resistance to disease, increased cold-climate hardiness, multiplied grain yield, and hugely increased the *glutentin* fraction of wheat protein that makes it so stretchable and kneadable for bread-making.

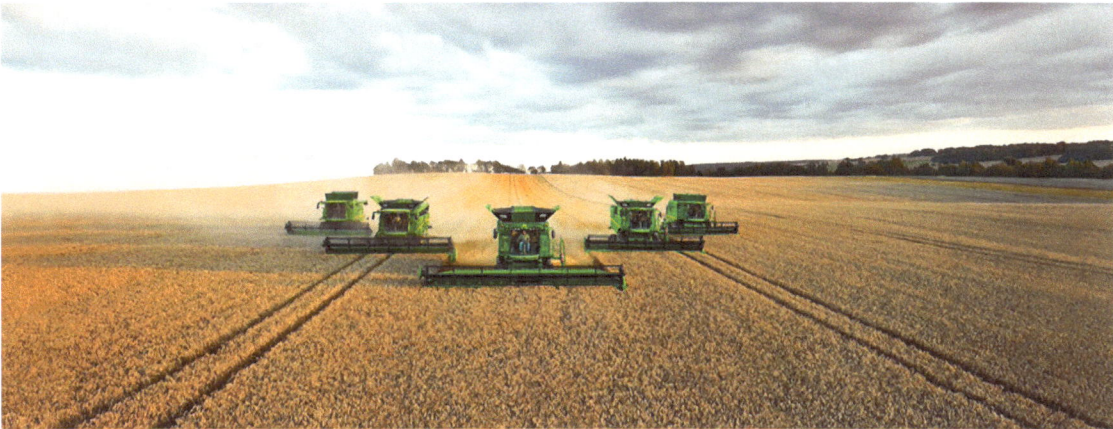

In the year 2000, the five largest wheat producers combined—the United States, Canada, Australia, the European Union, and Argentina—produced over 236.5 tons of wheat annually. As a species, we have become so wheat-dependent that world wheat production is perennial—wheat is being harvested in some part of the world in every month of the year. Only sixteen percent of wheat yield is fed to livestock world-wide—the bulk is consumed by humans. Grains—especially wheat—have been heavily subsidized by the government, resulting in astronomical production levels that continue to climb...alongside entreaties to eat more "whole grains" for health. USDA officials assert that whole grains reduce heart disease, may help with weight management, and are part of a healthy diet. These statements have never been supported by any legitimate scientific sources. We are expected to accept this because of the USDA's authority as a government bureaucracy.

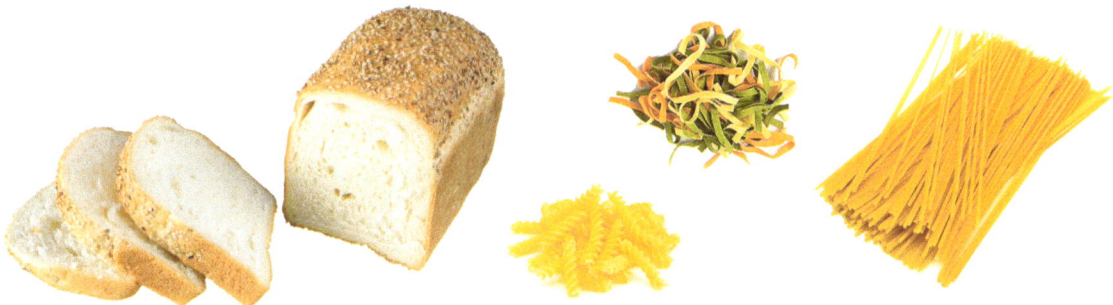

As you may have gathered by now, there's a great deal of effort and money involved in growing and marketing wheat. But we need to ask this one question: Is wheat—or any grain—*really* all that good for us?

Health Effects of a High-Wheat Diet

According to Dr. William Davis, M.D., author of *Wheat Belly: Lose the Wheat, Lose the Weight and Find Your Path Back to Health,* eating wheat is a dietary calamity. Recent research reveals that wheat, the so-called "staff of life," may harbor an unpleasant secret: Changes in wheat's biochemical profile through selective breeding and genetic manipulation may be responsible for our most common modern ills. The wheat and other grains of today bear little resemblance to grains of just decades ago, much less 10,000 years ago. A high-wheat diet has been linked to obesity, digestive diseases, arthritis, diabetes, heart disease, and dementia.

Blood Sugar and Insulin

Modern wheat is exceptionally high in *amylopectin-a,* a unique starch (unlike regular amylopectin found in rice and other grains) that is so quickly absorbed it rivals table sugar in the Glycemic Index (GI), a scale of sugar absorption and *glycemic* (blood sugar) increase as compared to glucose. Glucose has a GI of 100, so we compare other foods to it; the higher the number, the more the food raises blood sugar. (Glycemic Index & Glycemic Load are explained at length in "Health Concept #5—Dieting Strategies.")

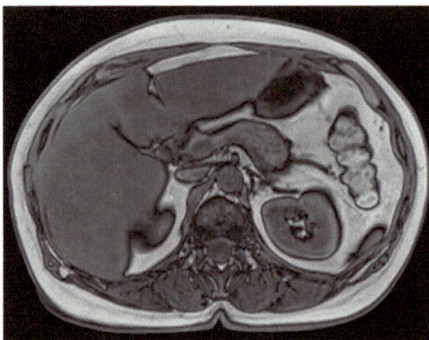

Abdomen with only subcutaneous fat   *Subcutaeous and **visceral** fat*

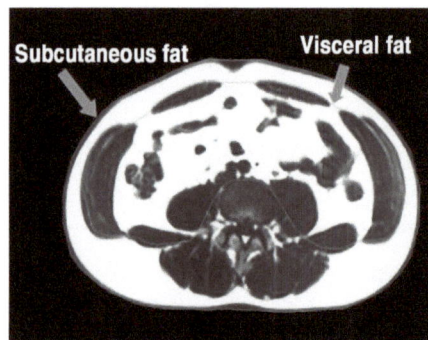

The surge in blood sugar and insulin that occurs with wheat consumption eventually causes an increase in *visceral* (internal) fat. This fat, mostly hidden from view (except with an MRI scan), makes the body more resistant to insulin and increases the risk for diabetes. Amylopectin-a also stimulates appetite—wheat-eaters typically eat 400 more Calories daily than their wheat-free counterparts.

Wheat Contains Unique Substances	
SUBSTANCE	**COMMENTS**
Amylopectin-a	a different form found in short-grain rice
Gluten	protein also found in barley and rye grains
Gliadin	a fraction of gluten
Phytic Acid	binds to minerals, making them unavailable to the body; also found in most other grains
Lectin	glycoprotein that binds to intestinal wall

Common table sugar (sucrose) has a GI 59; a slice of whole-wheat bread—72. Wheat *amylopectin-a* causes a significant insulin response, which as you will learn, is a pathway to hormone and enzyme profile disturbances that lead to inflammation and diseases such as metabolic syndrome, diabetes, heart-disease, arthritis, and cancer.

High Wheat Intake and *Lipidemia* (High Blood Fats)

Diets high in carbohydrates cause an increase in low-density lipoprotein (LDL) particles, the type of cholesterol that is most likely to lead to atherosclerosis and cardiovascular disease. Wheat dramatically increases the production of LDLs and VLDLs (*very* low-density lipoproteins), leading to heart disease. Researchers have known about this process for decades. What is the USDA *thinking* when they recommend eating more whole grains? You may be certain it is not your well-being.

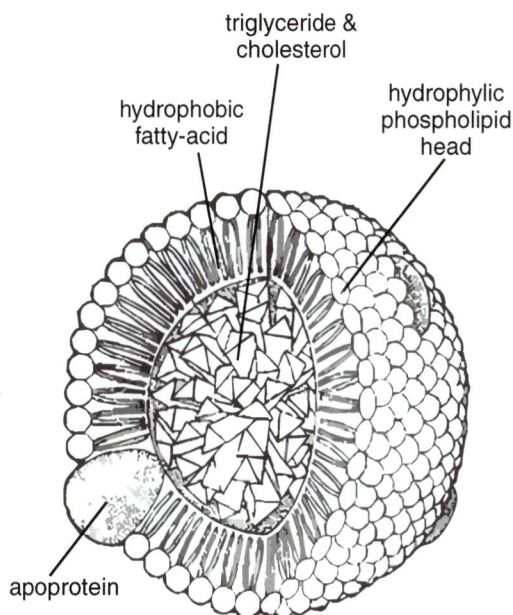

triglyceride & cholesterol

hydrophobic fatty-acid

hydrophylic phospholipid head

apoprotein

A typical cholesterol molecule of the phospholipid class

Body pH and Wheat

A wheat-rich diet shifts the body's chemistry to an acidic (low-pH) state. This condition, known as *acidosis*, leaches calcium from the bones, which then passes into the urine. Grains—and particularly wheat—account for 38% of the average American's acid load.

An acidic pH will also cause acid-reflux syndrome. Many doctors will tell patients to eat crackers to relieve acid-reflux pain—a sure way to move onto prescription histamine-2 receptor antacids. Instead, drink water and eat carrots, apples, or some other high-fiber produce to relieve acid-reflux and indigestion.

Gluten, Gliadin, and Lectin

The *gluten* protein (also found in barley and rye grains) in modern wheat is different in structure from the gluten in older forms of wheat. Humans have never before encountered the molecular structure of modern gluten in 10,000 years of consuming wheat.

While *celiac disease* caused by gluten sensitivity is a serious affliction of less than 1% of the U.S. population (3.2 million unfortunate souls), wheat harbors an unusual gluten sub-fraction called *gliadin* that affects many more people in subtle and insidious ways, who are not specifically gluten sensitive. Gliadin, like amylopectin-a, stimulates appetite. Wheat-eaters are hungry more often, and get sudden cravings—usually for more wheat products.

Eating wheat gluten and gliadin produce a euphoric "high" that release *exorphins*, morphine-like compounds in the brain. Wheat-eaters find that cutting wheat from the diet produces a kind of withdrawal that affects emotional stability, leading to anxiety, moodiness, and depression.

Lectins are *glycoproteins* (proteins bound to a carbohydrate) that can bind to the linings of human tissue, especially intestinal cells. Lectins disable cells in the GI tract, keeping them from repairing and rebuilding, contributing to "leaky-gut syndrome," in which the intestinal barrier erodes and allows unwanted molecules to pass into the bloodstream rather than being eliminated. Lectins (also known as *phytohemagglutinins*) are present in most legumes—especially in castor beans, which are toxic to most animals—but are more problematic in wheat because of the sheer volume most people eat daily.

New research suggests that those who consume large amounts of wheat on a daily basis (for example, dry cereal for breakfast, a sandwich for lunch, and pasta for dinner) may be more susceptible to dementia and Alzheimer's disease. There is a direct link among hyperinsulinism, diabetes, and Alzheimer's disease. Autopsies reveal that heavy wheat-eaters have more plaque build-up in their brains than those who abstain from wheat.

Moving Forward

If you are interested in reducing—or removing altogether—the wheat in your diet, do not make the mistake of buying and eating substitutes. While low-glycemic grains such as millet, quinoa, spelt, and kamut are excellent substitutes in small amounts, other grains will thwart your efforts to not only lose weight, but attain optimum health. Many "gluten-free" processed products on grocery shelves incorporate highly refined rice and root flours (tapioca, potato, and arrowroot) as substitutes. These flours are high-glycemic and will create some of the very conditions you may be hoping to avoid by eliminating wheat. The table on the next page may surprise you:

Carbohydrates in Various Flours			
FLOUR	AMOUNT	CARB GRAMS	GLYCEMIC INDEX
Almond flour	1 T	2	1
Arrowroot flour	1 T	7	85
Buckwheat flour	1 T	2	54
Coconut flour	1 T	0	0
Cornstarch	1 T	7	85
Green pea flour	1 T	6.0	50
Other nut flours	1 T	1.0	1
Peanut flour	1 T	2.0	1
Potato flour	1 T	11.0	90
Rice flour	1 T	6.0	95
Soy flour	1 T	2.0	25
Tapioca flour	1 T	6.5	93
Wheat flour (enriched white)	1 T	6.0	72
Wheat flour (whole wheat)	1 T	6.0	72

Corn

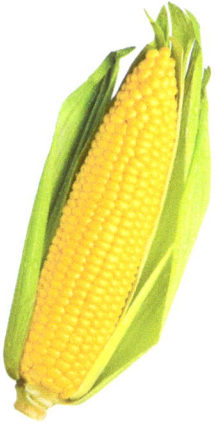

Modern corn has had a similar journey as wheat from small-eared, low-yield varieties of maize to the plump, sugar-filled corn varieties available today. The majority of corn grown in the United States is used in food processing, animal feed, and ethanol for vehicle fuel. There are very few varieties remaining for human consumption in its native form, with sweet white corn dominating commercial produce stands.

Food processing and manufacturing industries have found more than 4,200 uses for corn, with more being discovered daily. Processed corn products yield high-fructose corn syrup (HFCS), added to almost all processed packaged foods found on grocery store shelves. Corn starch is also a common food-additive. Bulk vitamin C (ascorbic acid) is manufactured from corn sugars. Corn products appear in fabrics, cosmetics, and baby powder. Varieties of corn are grown especially for livestock, to fatten them up in feed-lots across much of Nebraska and neighboring states. Corn is *everywhere.*

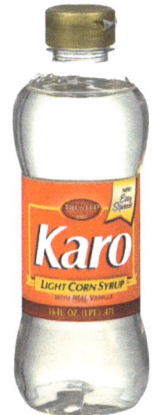

Is any of it nutritious? Unfortunately, corn has lost much of its flavor and nutrition through selective breeding, hybridization, and genetic modification. Corn is one of the first GMOs (genetically modified organisms) approved by the government for animal feed, then later for human consumption. It has modest nutritional value for vitamins and minerals, and is cultivated mostly for its sugar and starch content.

Commercial Uses for Corn	
EDIBLE	**NON-EDIBLE**
Acetic acid	Batteries
Amino acids	Blankets and bedding
Alcoholic beverages	Bookbinding
Antibiotics	Cardboard
Aspirin	Carpet tile
Baby food	Chalk
Bacon	Charcoal briquettes
Baked goods	Cleaners, detergents
Bakery products	Coatings on paper, wood, and metal
Baking powder	Color carrier for printing
Breadings, coatings, and batters	Cosmetics
Cake, cookie, dessert mixes	Crayons
Candies	Disposable diapers
Canned fruits, fruit fillings	Drink cups, plates, and cutlery
Caramel color	Dyes and inks
Carbonated and fruit beverages	Electroplating and galvanizing
Cereals	Fireworks
Cheese spreads	Food packaging
Chewing gum	Glues and adhesives
Citric acid	Industrial chemicals
Coffee whitener	Industrial filters
Condiments	Laminated building materials
Confections, chocolate	Leather tanning
Corn bread	Lubricants
Corn chips	Matches
Corn flakes	Metal plating
Cornmeal mixes	Ore and oil refining
Donuts	Organic solvents
Dried soups	Paints
Dusting for pizzas	Paper, recycled paper
English muffins	Pharmaceuticals
Enzymes	Plastics
Fermentation processes	Rayon
Food acids	Rubber tires
Food coloring	Shampoo
Fritters	Shaving cream
Frosting and icing	Shoe polish
Frozen and dried eggs	Sports and active wear

Commercial Uses for Corn, continued	
EDIBLE	**NON-EDIBLE**
Frozen pudding	Soaps and cleaners
Gravy mixes	Surgical dressings
Hams	Textiles
Hot dogs, bologna	Theatrical makeup
Hush puppies	Wallboard and wallpaper
Ice cream and sherbets	
Industrial sweetener	
Insecticides	
Instant breakfast foods	
Instant pudding mix	
Instant tea	
Jams, jellies, preserves	
Mannitol	
Marshmallows	
Meat products	
Muffins	
Pancake mixes	
Peanut butter	
Pet food	
Pickles and relishes	
Potato chips	
Powdered mixes	
Powdered sugar	
Precooked frozen foods	
Salad dressings	
Salt	
Sausage	
Seasoning mixes	
Snack foods	
Soups	
Spices	
Spoon bread	
Spray cooking oil	
Tomato sauces	
Vinegar	
Wine	
Worcestershire sauce	
Yeast	

Rice

Rice is a staple grain found almost everywhere in the world. Like wheat and corn, rice contains about 200 Calories per cup, and provides sustenance when little else is available, preventing starvation due to its ease of storage. Rice allergies are almost unknown, and rice does not cause digestive upsets or sensitivities. Rice is a poor source of protein and is an unwise choice for vegetarian food combining to make up complete proteins.

Rice does cause rises in blood sugar, with a glycemic index ranging from 50–75, depending on the variety of rice. Rice contains the starches *amylose* and *amylopectin.* Amylose is dominant in long-grain rice and is lower on the glycemic scale. Amylopectin dominates the starch in short-grain rice and forms sticky grains that pack well. Rounder and creamier high-amylopectin (or *glutinous*) rice is higher on the glycemic scale.

Common Rice Varieties

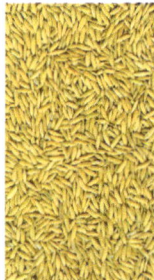

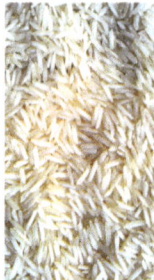

rough unpolished rice	brown long-grain rice	wild rice
white basmati rice	white fine basmati rice	white very fine basmati rice
brown short-grain rice	white short-grain rice	Vietnamese glutinous "mochigome" rice

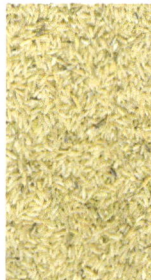

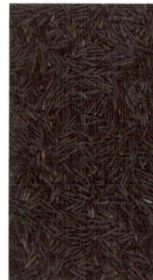

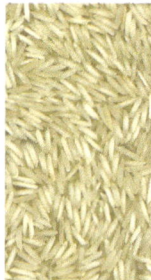

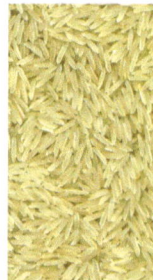

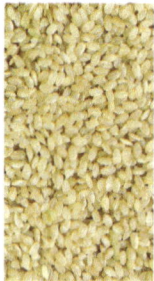

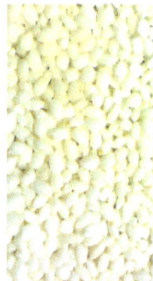

Rice Varieties Table		
RICE VARIETY	**GRAIN LENGTH**	**COMMENTS**
Arborio Rice	Short grain	usually used for risotto, it releases lots of amylopectin during cooking, so the finished dish is creamy and has a great soft mouth-feel
Basmati Rice	Long grain	aromatic (smells like popcorn when cooking), cooks up fluffy and separate. Brown basmati rice is the lowest-glycemic rice; tiny-grained basmati is around 50 GI.
Brown Rice	Medium grain	Only the hull is removed during processing; the bran is retained, resulting in more fiber and nutrients. Brown rice takes longer to cook than white rice because the outer layer is harder.
Converted Rice	Medium grain	This is rice that has been partially precooked, then dried, so it cooks more quickly. Vitamins from the bran are forced inside the rice grains during the conversion process. It's a good choice if you aren't picky about your rice quality; you are also guaranteed consistent results.
Instant Rice	Medium grain	is even more processed than converted rice; rehydrate it by adding hot water and letting it stand, covered, until tender
Jasmine Rice	Long grain	aromatic, but with more amylopectin than regular long grain rice, so it cooks up creamier than long grain
Long Grain White Rice	Long grain	Cooks up fluffy and separate.
Medium Grain Rice	Medium grain	has more amylopectin in the grains and a softer outer layer, so it releases starch during cooking and cooks up creamy.
Short Grain Rice	Short grain	has more amylopectin in the grains; releases lots of starch during cooking; sticky and creamy when cooked.
Vietnamese/Taiwanese *Mochigome* Glutinous Rice	Short-grain	is a very sticky and sweet rice grown and enjoyed in isolated regions of the far east, and shipped world-wide
Wehani Rice	Long grain	unpolished brown rice with a very sweet flavor. Cooks up fluffy and separate.
Wild Rice	Long grain	The seed of a native grass, this "rice takes longer to cook than brown rice and has a nutty flavor and chewy texture. It cooks up fluffy and separate, unless you cook it until it ruptures or the outer covering disintegrates, making it softer and less separate.

Grains are unnecessary in a healthy diet. There is *no nutrient in grains that cannot be supplied by other foods.* Produce, meats, dairy, and nuts and seeds contain the same nutrients found in grains, and in higher amounts. Use grains sparingly for flavor and variety, rather than using them to provide the bulk of your calories, and you *will* lose weight.

Protein

Of the three macro-nutrients, protein can arguably be considered the most important because of its role in so many biological systems. Protein is second only to oxygen and water to sustain life. The World Health Organization considers protein to be the most critical macro-nutrient to survival, and much human effort is expended to make certain that enough protein is available to everyone worldwide.

Proteins in animal tissue have many functions, as shown in the table below.

Function of Protein in Living Tissue	
PROTEIN CLASS	FUNCTION
Fibrous	Connective tissue, muscle, tendons; keratin in hair and nails
Globular	Hemoglobin, enzyme transporters
Structural	Collagen in skin and bone
Anabolic	Enzymes for combining and building molecules
Catalytic	Enzymes involved in breakdown processes
Hormonal	Integrated into hormones regulating physiological processes
Protective	Essential to antibody manufacture in immune response
Storage	Integrated with other substances and deposited for use later (short-term)
Regulation	Mediate cell processes through conjugation with other substances; binds to minerals to enable assimilation

Enough protein must be consumed daily to ensure *Nitrogen Equilibrium.* A "positive nitrogen balance" means getting at least 30 grams of *complete* protein daily for metabolic processes alone. "Negative nitrogen balance" occurs when daily intake is less than 30 grams, or less than optimum to prevent muscle wasting, reduced immune response, and other degenerative processes. Though the government guidelines for protein average 45–60 grams, protein requirements for individuals vary considerably, ranging from 30 to 200 grams. Decreased intake may be indicated for those with kidney disease; increased intake is required for dieters (as protein raises metabolism); athletes and burn victims have an elevated demand to replace protein lost due to tissue damage.

Protein Quality

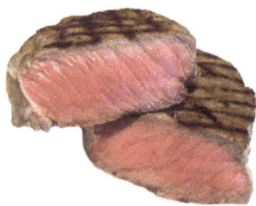

With few exceptions, complete proteins derive from animal-based foods and contain all of the amino acids in the proper ratios for sustaining human life. Incomplete proteins derive from plant-based foods, but combined together can provide enough high-quality (complete) protein necessary to health.

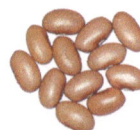

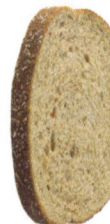

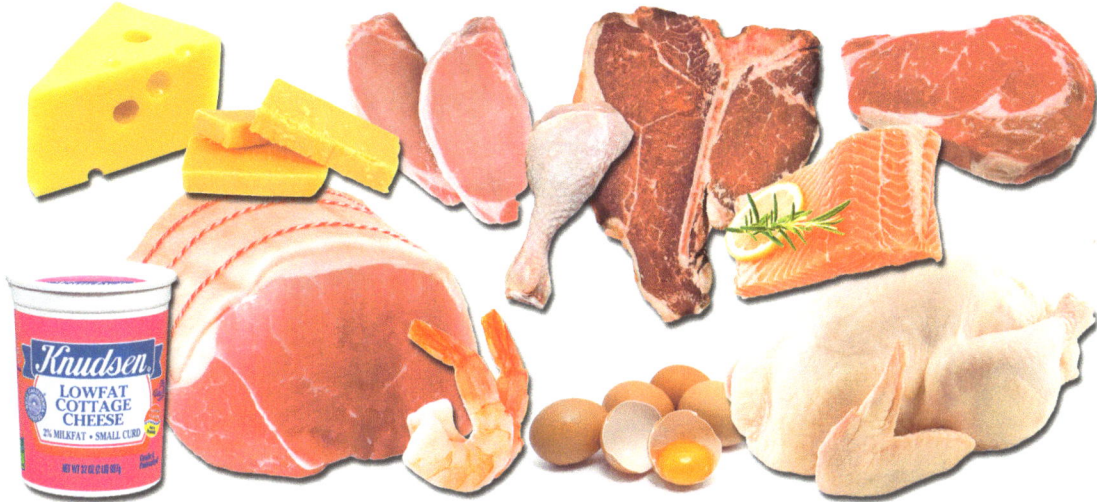

There are 10 essential amino acids. They are essential in that without daily intake, health declines and disease ensues.

Table of Common Amino Acids in Foods			
ESSENTIAL	**ABBREVIATION**	**NONESSENTIAL**	**ABBREVIATION**
Arginine (can be synthesized)	Arg	Glycine	Gly
Histidine (children)	His	Alanine	Ala
Isoleucine	Ile	Serine	Syr
Leucine	Leu	Cysteine	Cys
Lysine	Lys	Tyrosine	Tyr
Methionine	Met	Glutamine	Gln
Phenylalanine	Phe	Glutamic Acid	Glu
Tryptophan	Trp	Aspartic Acid	Asp
Threonine	Thr	Asparagine	Asn
Valine	Val	Proline	Pro

Humans are quite individual in their ability to metabolize and benefit from protein in food. Food allergies and malabsorption syndromes (such as gluten intolerance in celiac disease) affect protein absorption. Protein content in vegetable sources varies considerably. A fast and simple method for determining protein quality may be unattainable because of these factors. For decades, many systems of analyzing protein quality and assimilation have come and gone, only to be replaced by yet another system. Nevertheless, comparing protein quality across systems reveals common agreement as shown in the table on the next page.

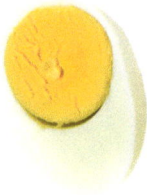

Protein Quality Table	
PROTEIN SOURCE	RATING
Eggs (whites)	1.0
Milk—human	0.9
Soybean isolate	0.9
Meats (beef, pork, poultry, seafood)	0.7–0.9
Milk—dairy (cow, goat, sheep)	0.7
Grains (wheat, corn, barley, oats)	0.4–0.7
Legumes (beans, peas, peanuts)	0.4–0.7
Potatoes	0.5
Rice	0.5

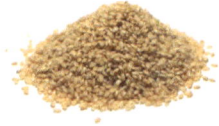

Combining Foods to Complement Amino Acids

Obtaining a full supply of complementary essential amino acids is of particular concern for vegans, specifically in obtaining the amino acid *lysine.* Fortunately, combining plant foods is can supply most of the essential complementary amino acids required by human physiology. Different foods with *limiting amino acids* (the amino acids that are the least abundant in the food) are consumed in a single meal to create a complete-protein complement. The body reassembles amino acids to create proteins for going about biological processes. To be effective, complementary limiting amino acids must be consumed in the *same* meal; they do not "wait around" for the complementary counterpart!

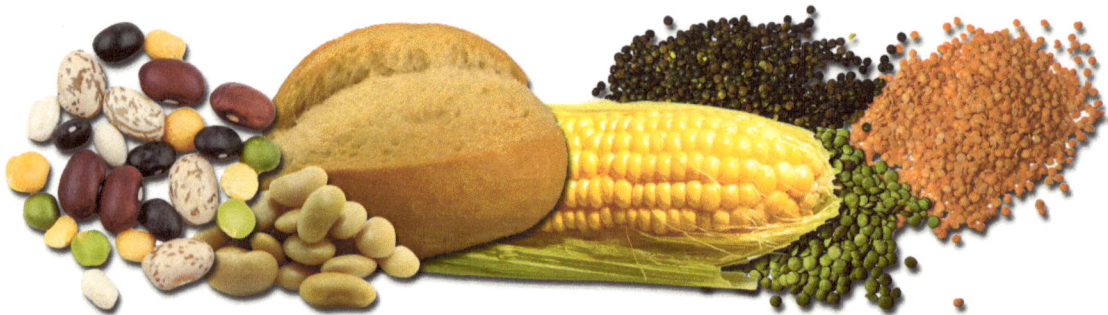

The "Limiting" Amino Acids (LAA)

- Lysine (of critical importance in vegan food combining)
- Isoleucine
- Methionine (of critical importance in vegan food combining)
- Threonine
- Tryptophan

Limiting Amino Acids in Food Groups				
FOOD GROUP	ISOLEUCINE	LYSINE	METHIONINE	TRYPTOPHAN	Low In...
Legumes	Yes	Yes	No	No	methionine, tryptophan
Grains	No	No	Yes	Yes	lysine, isoleucine
Together	Yes	Yes	Yes	Yes	none

Instructions

Using the following two Protein Tables (one for plant sources, the other for animal protein), fill out the Protein Sources Table in the Self-Assessment section that follows. Refer to your 24-Hour Food Journal from page 25 to complete that section.

Vegetable Protein Sources Table				
FOOD	QUANTITY	PROTEIN GRAMS	LIMITING AMINO ACID	%LAA
GRAINS				
Bread, French	1 slice	1.8	met	4
Bread, rye	1 slice	2.1	met	5
Bread, white enriched.	1 slice	2.0	met	5
Bread, whole wheat	1 slice	2.4	met	6
Corn, kernel	1 cup	3.8	met	11
Cornflakes	1 cup	2.0	met	5
Oatmeal	1 cup	4.8	met	13
Pasta noodles	1 cup	6.6	met	18
Popcorn	1 cup	1.8	met	4
Rice, brown	1 cup	3.8	met	10
Rice, white	1 cup	4.1	met	9
Tortilla, corn	1	1.5	met	4
Waffle	1 average	7.0	met	23
LEGUMES				
Beans, garbanzo, dry	4 oz	20.5	met	42
Beans, green	1 cup	2.0	met	5
Beans, lima	1 cup	9.2	-	39
Beans, soy	1 cup	22.0	met	53
Lentils	1 cup	15.6	met	15
Peanuts	4 oz	18.8	met	102
Peas, green	1 cup	8.6	met	7

Vegetable Protein Sources Table, continued				
FOOD	QUANTITY	PROTEIN GRAMS	LIMITING AMINO ACID	%LAA
NUTS				
Almonds	4 oz	14.6	met	54
Brazil nuts	4 oz	10.0	-	92
Pecans	4 oz	5.0	met	25
Pumpkin seeds	4 oz	20.3	met	202
Sunflower seeds	4 oz	17.4	met	19
Walnuts	4 oz	8.4	met	49
FRUITS				
Dates	10	2.2	met	7
Peach	1 medium	0.6	trp	2
Pear	1 medium	1.4	met	1
Persimmon	1 medium	0.8	met	1
VEGETABLES				
Asparagus	4 spears	2.2	met	1
Broccoli	1 cup	4.8	met	9
Cabbage	1 cup	0.9	met	2
Carrot	1 large	1.1	met	2
Cauliflower	1 cup	2.9	met	9
Celery	2 stalks	1.0	leu, phe, isl, val, thr	0
Cucumber	1 medium	0.9	met	1
Eggplant	1 cup	2.0	met	2
Lettuces	1 cup	0.7	leu, phe, isl, val, thr	0
Mushrooms, cooked	1 cup	3.3	lys, phe, thr	0
Onions, dry	1 cup	2.6	met	3
Peppers, bell	1 large	1.0	met	3
Potato, baked	1 medium	2.0	met	5
Pumpkin	1 cup	2.5	met	3
Radishes	10 medium	0.5	lys, phe, is	10
Spinach, cooked	1 cup	5.5	met	14
Squash, summer	1 cup	1.6	met	3
Squash, winter	1 cup	3.7	met	6
Sweet potato, baked	1 medium	4.8	met	6
Tomato	1 medium	1.6	-	2
Turnip greens	1 cup	3.0	met	8
Turnip root	1 cup	1.2	trp,leu,val,thr	0

Animal-Source and Mixed Foods Protein Table		
FOOD	QUANTITY	PROTEIN
DAIRY		
Butter	.5 oz (1 T)	0
Cheese, American	1 oz	6.50
Cheese, cheddar	1 oz	7.40
Cheese, cottage, low-fat	4 oz	14.00
Cheese, cottage, nonfat	4 oz	14.00
Cheese, cottage, regular	4 oz	14.00
Cheese, cream	1 oz	2.20
Cheese, jack	1 oz	6.94
Cheese, mozzarella, part-skim	1 oz	7.79
Cheese, Parmesan, dry	1 oz	4.16
Cheese, Swiss	1 oz	8.06
Cream, half-and-half	1 oz	0.88
Cream, heavy	1 oz	0.61
Cream, substitute	1 oz	0.40
Egg	1 large	6.00
Egg Beaters	2 oz	6.00
Ice cream	8 oz	4.80
Ice milk	8 oz	5.16
Milk, 2% fat	8 oz	8.12
Milk, buttermilk	8 oz	8.10
Milk, condensed sweet	8 oz	24.80
Milk, nonfat	8 oz	8.40
Milk, whole 4% fat	8 oz	8.50
Yogurt, plain low-fat	8 oz	11.90
Yogurt, plain nonfat	8 oz	12.00
Yogurt, plain whole-milk	8 oz	7.88
MEATS		
Beef, dry chipped	3 oz	29.10
Beef, ground supreme-lean	4 oz	34.19
Beef, jerky	1 piece	4.20
Beef, roast lean	4 oz	36.10
Beef, short-ribs	4 oz	27.72
Beef, steak porterhouse	4 oz	29.00
Beef, steak round	4 oz	43.99
Beef, steak sirloin	4 oz	28.93
Beef, steak T-bone	4 oz	28.66

Animal-Source and Mixed Foods Protein Table, continued		
FOOD	QUANTITY	PROTEIN
Beef, tenderloin strip	4 oz	29.53
Beef, veal cutlet	4 oz	37.94
Franks, all meat	1	7.00
Franks, turkey	1	5.80
Lamb, chops	4 oz	30.86
Lamb, leg roast	4 oz	31.21
Lunch meat, bologna, meat	1 slice	2.70
Lunch meat, bologna, turkey	1 slice	3.90
Lunch meat, deviled ham	½ can	9.00
Lunch meat, olive loaf	1 slice	3.40
Lunch meat, pickle loaf	1 slice	3.30
Lunch meat, salami, beef	1 slice	3.40
Lunch meat, turkey ham	1 slice	3.90
Lunch meat, turkey pastrami	1 slice	5.20
Pepperoni	1 slice	1.20
Pork , ham cured	4 oz	28.56
Pork, bacon	1 slice	1.60
Pork, chops	4 oz	33.60
Pork, roast	4 oz	20.14
Pork, sausage	4 oz	22.32
Pork, sirloin	4 oz	31.20
Pork, spare-ribs	8 med	23.72
Rabbit	4 oz	35.31
Spam	1 oz	3.90
Venison	4 oz	33.71
POULTRY		
Chicken thigh fried	1	16.60
Chicken, breast fried	½-piece	28.80
Chicken, breast no skin	½-piece	26.70
Chicken, breast w/skin	½-piece	29.20
Chicken, drum fried	1	13.20
Chicken, drum no skin	1	12.50
Chicken, drum w/skin	1	14.10
Chicken, gizzards	3.5 oz	27.20
Chicken, ground breast	4 oz	32.00
Chicken, livers	3.5 oz	24.40
Chicken, thigh no skin	1	13.50

Animal-Source and Mixed Foods Protein Table, continued		
FOOD	QUANTITY	PROTEIN
Chicken, thigh w/skin	1	15.50
Duck, no skin	4 oz	26.86
Goose, no skin	4 oz	33.14
Turkey, dark meat	4 oz	32.69
Turkey, ground, 10% fat	4 oz	34.00
Turkey, white meat	4 oz	34.17
SEAFOOD		
Bass	4 oz	21.43
Caviar, sturgeon	1 tsp	2.70
Clams, canned	4 oz	7.90
Clams, fresh	9 small	14.00
Cod	4 oz	19.95
Crab, canned	4 oz	13.90
Crab, fresh	4 oz	19.60
Crab, fried	4 oz	10.70
Fish cakes	4 oz	25.24
Fish fillets, breaded	4 oz	11.00
Fish sticks, fried	5 sticks	19.00
Haddock	4 oz	20.75
Halibut	4 oz	23.70
Herring, pickled	3.5 oz	20.00
Lobster	1 med. tail	20.00
Mackerel	4 oz	24.66
Mussels, steamed	4 oz	16.46
Oysters, canned	4 oz	10.10
Oysters, fried	4 oz	23.20
Perch	4 oz	21.50
Red Snapper	4 oz	22.45
Salmon, pink canned	4 oz	22.50
Salmon, pink fresh	4 oz	25.50
Salmon, sockeye canned	4 oz	23.35
Sardines, canned in oil	1 oz	6.80
Scallops, fresh	4 oz	17.35
Scallops, fried	4 oz	20.57
Shrimp, boiled	4 oz	20.53
Shrimp, fried	4 oz	23.20
Sole	4 oz	18.95

Animal-Source and Mixed Foods Protein Table, continued		
FOOD	QUANTITY	PROTEIN
Swordfish	4 oz	24.38
Trout, rainbow	4 oz	23.54
Tuna, albacore in oil	6.5 oz	50.60
Tuna, albacore in water	6.5 oz	51.50
Tuna, light in oil	6.5 oz	46.90
Tuna, light in water	6.5 oz	45.00
PROCESSED FOODS		
Banquet beef pie	8 oz	16.30
Banquet chicken pie	8 oz	16.30
Banquet enchilada, beef	12 oz	17.00
Banquet enchilada, cheese	12 oz	18.40
Banquet fish dinner	8.75 oz	19.30
Banquet macaroni and cheese	12 oz	13.30
Banquet meatloaf dinner	10.75 oz	19.00
Banquet meatloaf, Man Pleaser	19 oz	35.60
Banquet Mexican combination	12 oz	22.00
Banquet Salisbury steak	11 oz	18.10
Banquet Salisbury steak, Man Pleaser	19 oz	37.70
Banquet turkey dinner	11 oz	23.40
Banquet turkey, Man Pleaser	19 oz	39.30
Banquet veal Parmagian	11 oz	20.60
Campbell's Beans and Franks	8 oz	15.00
Celeste pizza, cheese	¼ pizza	14.43
Celeste pizza, deluxe	¼ pizza	16.20
Celeste pizza, pepperoni	¼ pizza	16.30
Celeste pizza, sausage	¼ pizza	16.00
Chef Boyardee Beefaroni	7.5 oz	8.00
Chef Boyardee Ravioli, beef	7.5 oz	7.00
Chili con Carne w/beans	1 cup	18.00
Chili con Carne, no beans	1 cup	26.00
Dinner Classics beef short ribs	10.5 oz	26.00
Dinner Classics chicken/noodles	12 oz	27.00
Dinner Classics Salisbury steak	11.5 oz	21.00
Dinner Classics sirloin roast	11 oz	29.00
Dinner Classics turkey/dressing	11.25 oz	19.00
Egg rolls, La Choy	4	3.80
Gravy, beef canned	½ can	5.40

Animal-Source and Mixed Foods Protein Table, continued		
FOOD	QUANTITY	PROTEIN
Gravy, brown from mix	4 oz	1.00
Gravy, chicken canned	½ can	2.80
Gravy, chicken from mix	4 oz	1.30
Hamburger Helper beef noodle	⅕ pkg.	20.00
Hamburger Helper beef Romanoff	⅕ pkg.	21.00
Hamburger Helper cheeseburger mac	⅕ pkg.	21.00
Hamburger Helper chili tomato	⅕ pkg.	19.00
Hamburger Helper hash	⅕ pkg.	18.00
Hamburger Helper lasagna	⅕ pkg.	19.00
Hamburger Helper pizza bake	⅕ pkg.	20.00
Hamburger Helper potato Stroganoff	⅕ pkg.	18.00
Hamburger Helper potatoes au gratin	⅕ pkg.	18.00
Hamburger Helper rice oriental	⅕ pkg.	18.00
Hamburger Helper spaghetti	⅕ pkg.	20.00
Hamburger Helper stew	⅕ pkg.	18.00
Hamburger Helper tamale pie	⅕ pkg.	4.00
Hash, corned beef	6 oz	24.00
Le Menu sliced turkey	11.25 oz	28.00
Macaroni and cheese, Kraft	6 oz	9.00
Noodle Roni Parmesano, dry	1.2 oz	5.00
Pork and beans	6 oz	11.00
Soup, bean canned	1 cup	8.00
Soup, chicken canned	1 cup	4.00
Soup, cream of...canned	1 cup	7.00
Soup, noodle; barley; rice	1 cup	6.00
Soup, split pea canned	1 cup	8.00
Soup, vegetable beef canned	1 cup	6.00
Spaghetti and meat sauce canned	1 cup	13.00
Stew, beef canned	1 cup	15.00
Stouffer's French bread pizza, cheese	5.13 oz	10.00
Stouffer's French bread pizza, deluxe	5.13 oz	15.00
Stouffer's French bread pizza, peprni.	5.13 oz	12.00
Stouffer's lasagna	10.5 oz	28.00
Stovetop bread stuffing	1 cup	6.00
Swanson beef dinner	15 oz	29.00
Swanson beef lasagna	12.25 oz	25.00
Swanson beef, Hungry Man	17 oz	44.00

Animal-Source and Mixed Foods Protein Table, continued		
FOOD	**QUANTITY**	**PROTEIN**
Swanson fried chicken dinner	15 oz	24.00
Swanson ham dinner	10 oz	19.00
Swanson Salisbury steak, Hungry Man	16 oz	23.00
Swanson turkey dinner	16 oz	27.00
Swanson turkey, Hungry Man	18.75 oz	48.00
Swanson veal parmagiana	11 oz	20.60
Tamales, canned	1	3.50
Tuna Helper	⅕ pkg.	14.00
Van de Kamps enchiladas, beef	4	16.00
Van de Kamps enchiladas, chicken	7.5 oz	14.00
Van de Kamps enchiladas, shred. beef	6 oz	12.00
Van de Kamps fillet o' fish	12 oz	25.00
Van de Kamps fish and chips	5 oz	13.00
Van de Kamps microwave sole	5 oz	16.00
FAST FOOD		
Arby's Club sandwich	1	30.00
Arby's Ham and cheese sandwich	1	33.00
Arby's Roast beef sandwich	1	22.00
Arby's Super roast beef sandwich	1	30.00
Arby's Turkey sandwich	1	28.00
Burger King Apple pie	1	2.00
Burger King Chicken Tenders	6 pieces	20.00
Burger King Chocolate shake	1	8.00
Burger King Double Beef Whopper	1	51.00
Burger King French fries, regular	1 pak	3.00
Burger King Onion rings	1 pak	3.00
Burger King Whopper with cheese	1	33.00
Carl's Jr. California Roast Beef sandwich	1	25.00
Carl's Jr. Famous Star burger	1	24.00
Carl's Jr. Filet of Fish sandwich	1	20.00
Carl's Jr. French fries, regular	1	3.00
Carl's Jr. Onion rings	1 pak	5.00
Carl's Jr. Super Star burger	1	43.00
Dairy Queen Buster Bar	1	10.00
Dairy Queen Cheese dog, super	1	26.00
Dairy Queen Cheeseburger	1	18.00
Dairy Queen Chili dog	1	13.00

Animal-Source and Mixed Foods Protein Table, continued		
FOOD	QUANTITY	PROTEIN
Dairy Queen Chili dog, super	1	23.00
Dairy Queen Dilly Bar	1	4.00
Dairy Queen Hamburger	1	13.00
Dairy Queen Hamburger, big	1	27.00
Dairy Queen Hamburger, super	1	53.00
Dairy Queen Hot dog	1	11.00
Dairy Queen Shake, large	1	22.00
Domino's Pizza 12" pepperoni	2 slices	20.00
Domino's Pizza 12" cheese	2 slices	18.00
Domino's Pizza 16" cheese	2 slices	24.00
Domino's Pizza 16" pepperoni	2 slices	24.00
Jack In The Box Apple turnover	1	4.00
Jack In The Box Cheeseburger	1	16.00
Jack In The Box Chicken Supreme sandwich	1	31.00
Jack In The Box Chocolate shake	1	11.00
Jack In The Box Fish Supreme sandwich	1	17.00
Jack In The Box French fries, regular	1	2.00
Jack In The Box Hamburger	1	13.00
Jack In The Box Jumbo Jack	1	28.00
Jack In The Box Jumbo Jack with cheese	1	32.00
Jack In The Box Onion rings	1 pak	5.00
Jack In The Box Super Taco	1	12.00
Jack In The Box Taco, regular	1	8.00
KFC Coleslaw	1	9.00
KFC Extra-crispy breast	1 piece	18.00
KFC Extra-crispy drumstick	1 pice	13.00
KFC Kentucky Fries	1 pak	5.00
KFC Kentucky Nuggets	6	17.00
KFC Original Recipe breast	1 piece	20.00
KFC Original Recipe drumstick	1 piece	14.00
KFC Potatoes and gravy	1	2.00
Long John Silver's Batter-fried fish dinner	1	17.00
Long John Silver's Batter-fried fish	1 piece	13.00
Long John Silver's Chicken Nugget dinner	6-piece	23.00
Long John Silver's Chicken Plank	1	9.00
Long John Silver's Fried fish dinner	3-piece	47.00
Long John Silver's Fryes	1 pak	4.00

Animal-Source and Mixed Foods Protein Table, continued		
FOOD	QUANTITY	PROTEIN
Long John Silver's Hushpuppies	2	3.00
McDonald's Big Mac	1	25.00
McDonald's Chicken McNuggets	6	19.00
McDonald's Chocolate shake	1	10.00
McDonald's Egg McMuffin	1	19.00
McDonald's Filet o' Fish sandwich	1	14.00
McDonald's French fries, regular	1	3.00
McDonald's Hamburger	1	13.00
McDonald's McDLT	1	30.00
McDonald's Quarter-pounder with cheese	1	30.00
Pizza Hut beef, thick	½—10"	38.00
Pizza Hut beef, thin	½—10"	29.00
Pizza Hut cheese, thick	½—10"	34.00
Pizza Hut cheese, thin	½—10"	25.00
Pizza Hut pepperoni, thick	½—10"	31.00
Pizza Hut pepperoni, thin	½—10"	23.00
Pizza Hut sausage, thin	½—10"	27.00
Pizza Hut supreme, thick	½—10"	36.00
Pizza Hut supreme, thin	½—10"	27.00
Pizza Hut sausage, thick	½—10"	36.00
Taco Bell Bean burrito	1	15.00
Taco Bell Beef burrito	1	30.00
Taco Bell Beefy tostada	1	19.00
Taco Bell Burrito Supreme	1	21.00
Taco Bell Combination burrito	1	21.00
Taco Bell Enchirito	1	19.00
Taco Bell Pintos n' Cheese	1	13.00
Taco Bell Taco, regular	1	12.00
Taco Bell Tostada	1	9.00
Wendy's Chicken sandwich	1	25.00
Wendy's Chili con carne	1	19.00
Wendy's Chocolate shake	1	9.00
Wendy's Double hamburger	1	41.00
Wendy's French fries, regular	1 pak	4.00
Wendy's Taco salad	1	23.00
Wendy's Triple cheeseburger	1	72.00

Instructions

Use the Protein Tables on the previous pages to fill in your Protein Sources Table below, then answer the questions in the Self-Assessment section that follows to evaluate your protein intake.

Protein Sources Table			
MEAL	PROTEIN GRAMS FROM PLANT SOURCES	% LAA	PROTEIN GRAMS FROM ANIMAL/MIXED SOURCES
BREAKFAST			
LUNCH			
DINNER			
SNACKS			
ADD UP THE %LAA OF PLANT-SOURCE PROTEIN →		_____	
THEN DIVIDE BY THE NUMBER OF SOURCES →		_____	This is Your Total %LAA of Plant Protein Consumed

Total Percent of Limiting Amino Acids (%LAA) of Plant-Source Protein divided by the *Number* of Plant Protein Sources = Total %LAA

Self-Assessment

1. Referring to your Food Journal, what is your daily average of protein from all sources?

   _____

2. Are you in "positive nitrogen balance" or "negative nitrogen balance" for the day?

   _____

3. Do you engage in body-building or other activities that require an increased protein intake?

   _____

4. Is your protein intake satisfactory, or is there room for improvement?

   _____

5. Fill out the Protein Sources Table that follows, referring to your Food Journal that you completed earlier. Calculate how much protein came from animal sources, and how much came from plant sources. Then, calculate the percentage of the total Limiting Amino Acids (%LAA) from plant sources you consumed. You can calculate this by *adding* the individual percentages of Limiting Amino Acids for *each* plant source, then *dividing this total* by the *number* of plant-protein sources to arrive at the total %LAA consumed on this day.

6. How close to 100% of the Limiting Amino Acids from plant protein sources, did you achieve?

   _____

7. Do you think you could or would ever want to adopt a vegetarian lifestyle, or do you feel your best consuming animal protein?

   _____

Protein Deficiency Diseases

Though rare in the United States, protein deficiency worldwide is a serious problem. Progression of deficiency states result in varying degrees of disease. In countries such as Rwanda and Bangladesh, for example, severe protein deficiency (starvation) may result in a condition known as *marasmus,* featuring profound muscle wasting with no body fat. A less severe form of inadequate protein intake called *kwashiorkor* results in negative nitrogen balance leading to fluid in the abdominal cavity (acites).

Conversely, very high-protein diets (exceeding 100 grams daily) can potentially cause a vast array of metabolic problems. High-protein diets are hard on the kidneys, so water intake must be increased with more protein consumption. However, high water intake causes mineral losses through increased urination and the necessity for mineral and vitamin supplementation. High-protein diets are inadvisable without expertise in nutrition or consulting with a nutritionist or biochemist.

Dietary Fats (Lipids)

Fats may carry the most Calories (9 Calories per gram), but they are necessary to good health, so reducing or cutting fat out of your diet is a misguided strategy for weight control.

There are three major classes of dietary fats: polyunsaturated (also sometimes referred to as omega-6, but also includes omega-3s), monounsaturated (omega-9), and saturated (omega-6 and beyond). The "omega" designation indicates the position of the endmost (last)) double bond on the triglyceride molecule. Unfortunately, fats have acquired a great deal of controversy and have been vilified in the mainstream media in recent decades. It seems that no one can agree. But biochemists, physiologists, and nutritionists have researched lipids extensively and have discovered some important facts about fats that may surprise you.

Unsaturated Fat (Triglyceride) Molecule

Oleic Acid

Saturated Fat (Triglyceride) Molecule

Stearic Acid

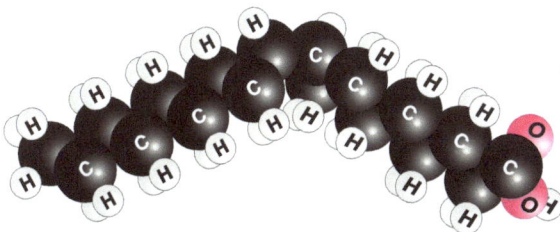

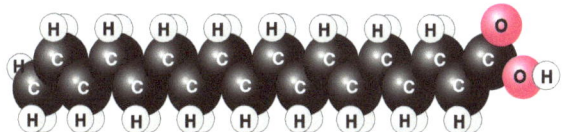

Unsaturated Fat (Triglyceride) Molecule

Linoleic Acid

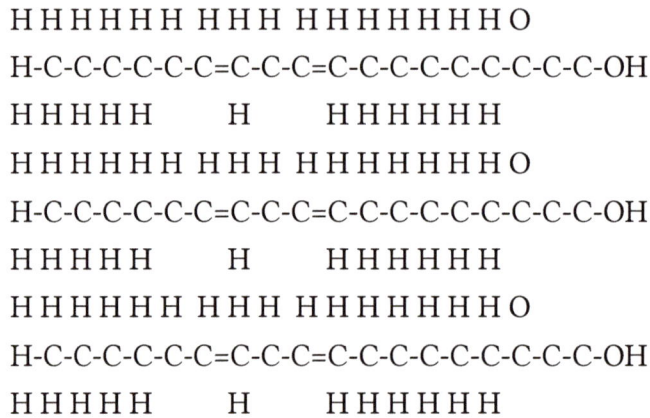

```
H H H H H H   H H H   H H H H H H H O
H-C-C-C-C-C-C=C-C-C=C-C-C-C-C-C-C-C-C-OH
  H H H H H       H         H H H H H H

H H H H H H   H H H   H H H H H H H O
H-C-C-C-C-C-C=C-C-C=C-C-C-C-C-C-C-C-C-OH
  H H H H H       H         H H H H H H

H H H H H H   H H H   H H H H H H H O
H-C-C-C-C-C-C=C-C-C=C-C-C-C-C-C-C-C-C-OH
  H H H H H       H         H H H H H H
```

Saturated Fat (Triglyceride) Molecule

Palmitic Acid

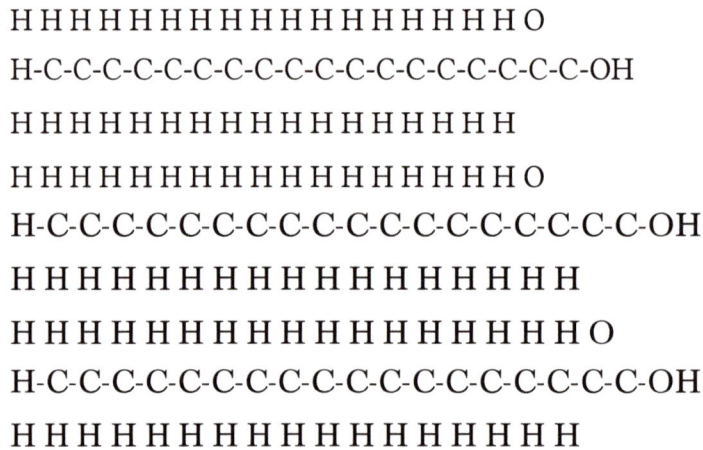

```
H H H H H H H H H H H H H H H H H O
H-C-C-C-C-C-C-C-C-C-C-C-C-C-C-C-C-C-OH
  H H H H H H H H H H H H H H H H H

H H H H H H H H H H H H H H H H H O
H-C-C-C-C-C-C-C-C-C-C-C-C-C-C-C-C-C-OH
  H H H H H H H H H H H H H H H H H

H H H H H H H H H H H H H H H H H O
H-C-C-C-C-C-C-C-C-C-C-C-C-C-C-C-C-C-OH
  H H H H H H H H H H H H H H H H H
```

Not all fats are equal! Some fats *cause* cellular damage, while other fats *protect* cells from damage. Beneficial fats come from all three groups, and so do damaging fats. So, how do we tell the difference?

Bad Lipids

As mentioned earlier, processed, chemically-extracted polyunsaturated fats in the form of grain seed oils found in processed foods are health destroying. These fats cause *free-radical* damage leading to disease states. (Free radicals are damaged atoms or molecules with unpaired electrons, making them very bioreactive.) Refined and processed polyunsaturates accelerate aging, and promote inflammatory processes leading to cancer, heart disease, joint disease, and type-2 diabetes.

Hydrogenated fats have been artificially saturated to stabilize them, and are known to cause heart disease and other metabolic ills, such as insulin resistance, which can lead to type-2 diabetes. Hydrogenated fats raise LDLs (low-density lipoproteins—so-called "bad" cholesterol) and lower HDLs (high-density lipoproteins—"good" cholesterol). Imitation cheese, margarine, and solid vegetable fats used in frying and baking are three of the most notorious hydrogenated fats. Avoid these fats completely if you want to remain healthy!

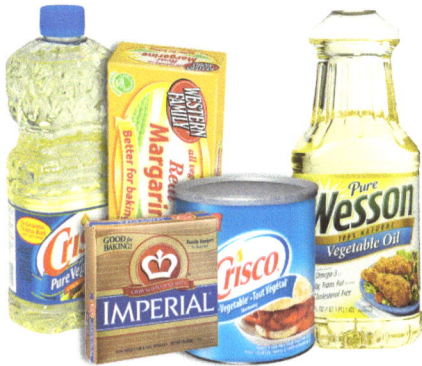

THIS JUST IN... Not all LDLs are bad! Pattern-a LDL is buoyant and does not become part of arterial epithelial plaque. Pattern-b LDL sinks and integrates with the plaque. High triglycerides influence the LDL pattern class, in that higher triglycerides translate to more pattern-b LDL. Pattern-b LDL (small dense molecules) correlate with a *high-carbohydrate diet*.

Cholesterol is Critical for Hormone Production

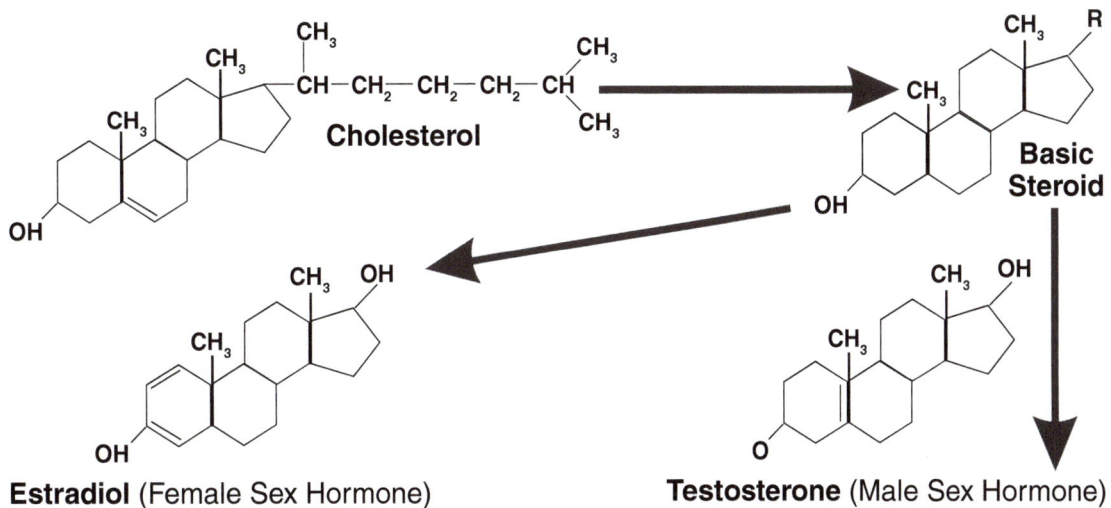

Cholesterol

Basic Steroid

Estradiol (Female Sex Hormone)

Testosterone (Male Sex Hormone)

Many people believe that saturated fats from meat are unhealthful. In actuality, meats contain about 50% saturated fats; the other 50% is unsaturated. The health-damaging effects of eating commercially-produced meat is directly attributable to a specific polyunsaturated omega-6 fatty acid called *arachidonic acid.* This fatty acid promotes inflammation. Arachidonic acid is so high in commercial meat and dairy because of the animals' high-grain diet, which is not natural to them. Consequently, feed-lot raised beef and pork, and commercial dairy animals produce excess arachidonic acid in their tissues, and pass it on to you. You will also significantly raise your own production of arachidonic acid when you eat a high refined-carbohydrate diet (notably grain products).

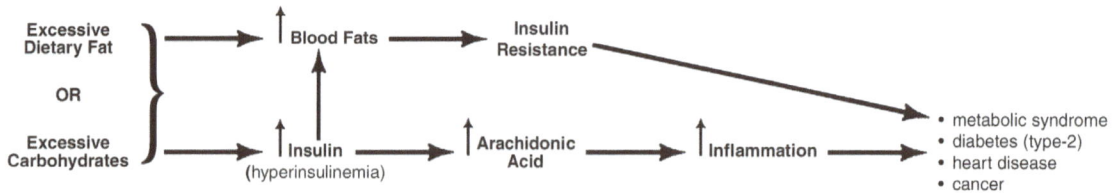

Good Lipids

Polyunsaturated Fatty Acids

Modest amounts of polyunsaturated fats from whole nuts and seeds are part of a healthful diet. Wheat germ and whole grains also contain small amounts of these essential oils. Polyunsaturated fats rancidify very easily, and create free radicals when heated above 150 °F. It is best to keep foods high in these oils refrigerated until eaten. Excess intake of polyunsaturated fats (a class of omega-6 fats) is pro-inflammatory, leading to disease states.

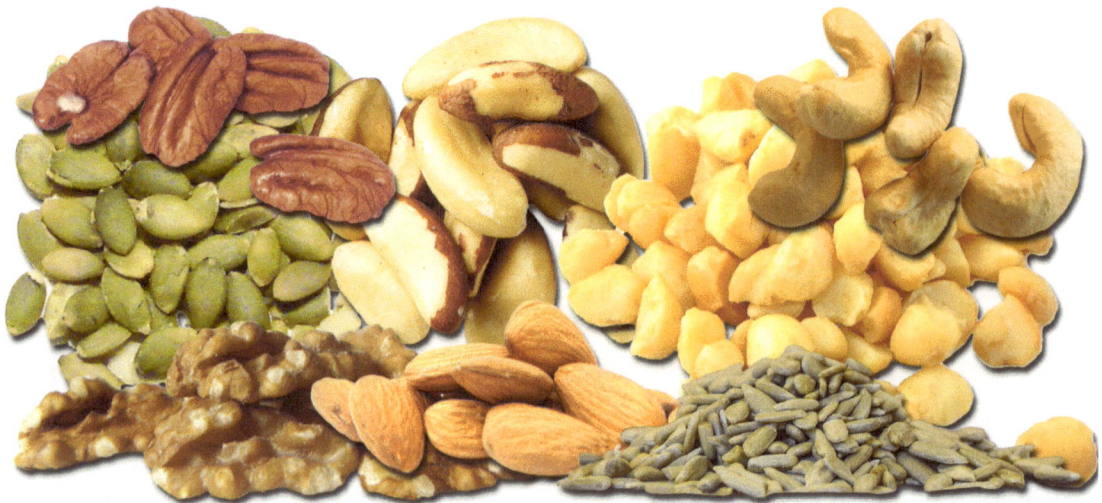

Omega-3 Fatty Acids

Omega-3 fats from cold-water fish, krill, and shellfish contain both polyunsaturated and saturated fats. They are incredibly beneficial to health, but are typically low in the average American diet. Omega-3 fats reduce inflammation, and help ameliorate the pro-inflammatory effect of excess polyunsaturates of the omega-6 class. While flaxseed and Sacha Inchi oils have been marketed as a healthy omega-3 fat especially for vegans, the body must convert the healthful omega-6 α-linolenic acid (ALA) in these oils to the omega-3s eicosapentaenoic acid (EPA) and docosahexaenoic acid (DHA), as found natively in fish oils. The human body is not very efficient at this conversion.

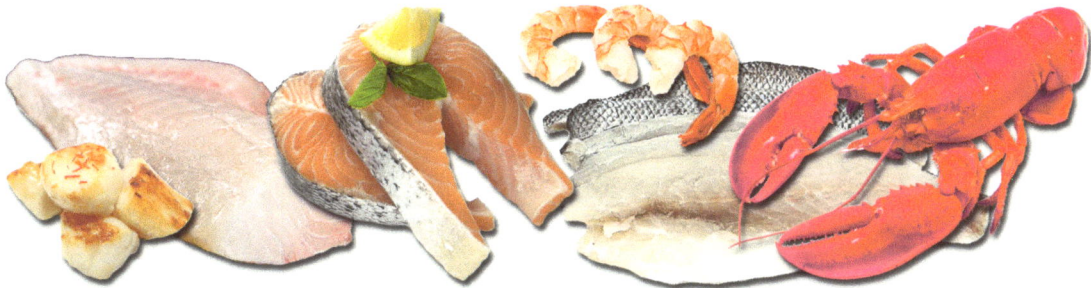

Monounsaturated Fatty Acids (Omega-9s)

Beneficial fats also include monounsaturated oils derived from olives, avocados, walnuts, macadamias, and almonds. Monounsaturated oils reduce serum cholesterol with consistent intake. Whole cold-pressed monounsaturated oils also contain saturated and polyunsaturated oils, providing a healthful balance of all three classes of dietary fats. Monounsaturated oils are the foundation of the often-praised Mediterranean diet.

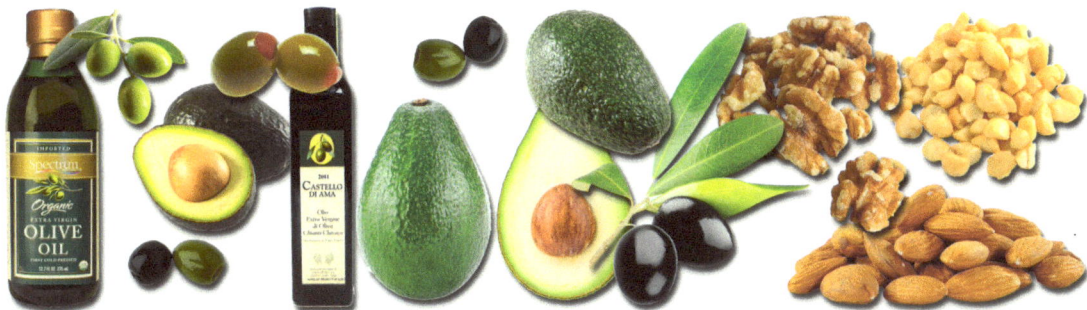

Saturated Fatty Acids

Saturated fats are not intrinsically bad for human heath. Short- and medium-chain saturated fats—as found in butter fat, tropical oils, and human breast milk—are essential to health. In fact, saturated fats are essential for many biological processes, are crucial to blood vessel wall integrity, are a component of nerve cell sheaths (myelin), and are vital to hormone production. Avoiding all saturated fats will increase susceptibility to a particular kind of stroke (intraparenchymal hemorrhage), and cause many other health problems.

Saturated fats from grass-fed beef and range-fed pork and poultry, and some vegetable sources, are the most healthful. Fats from range-fed animals is very low in arachidonic acid—and high in omega-3 fats—and do not promote inflammation or disease states as feed-lot raised meats do. Dairy products and eggs from range-fed animals are also lower in inflammatory fatty acids than the products from grain-fed dairy animals.

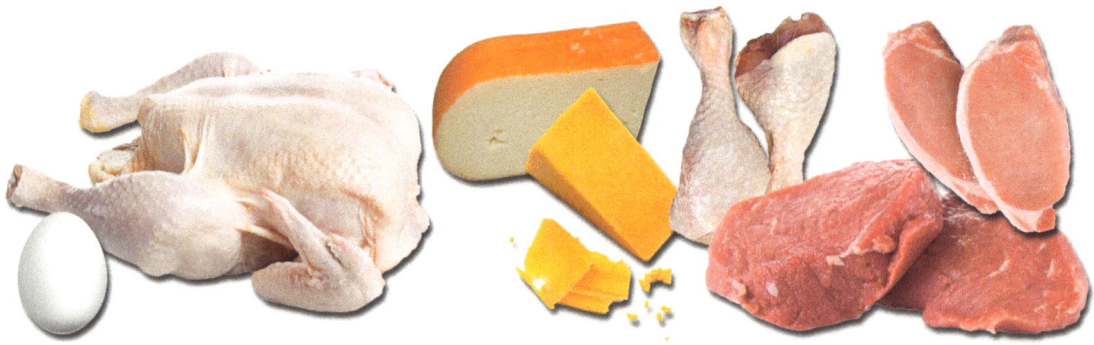

Tropical Oils

Researchers have discovered that two of the most saturated fats known—coconut and palm oils—are some of the most beneficial to health. Coconut and palm oils do not go rancid at room temperature and exposure to air—as polyunsaturates do—and are not subject to free-radical damage when heated, which makes them ideal for cooking.

Short- and medium-chain triglycerides—rather than the long-chain triglycerides that make up most other dietary fats—comprise coconut and palm oils, which are not stored as adipose tissue (body fat), but burned for fuel. Tropical oils are *thermogenic* (create heat) so they raise metabolism while inhibiting the liver's formation and storage of fat. These properties make tropical oils useful in weight reduction.

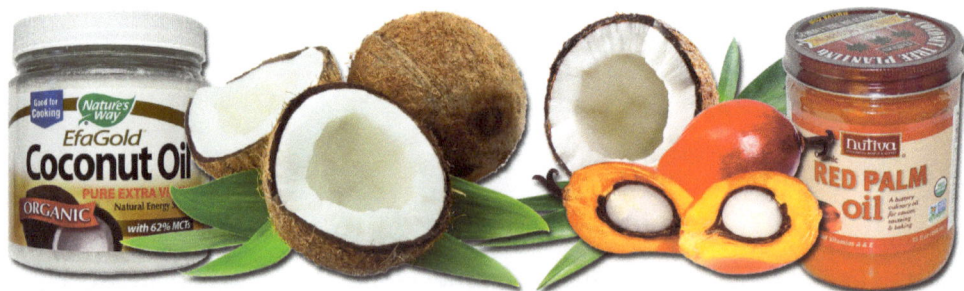

Dairy Fats (butterfat)

Dairy products have taken a media beating in recent years, primarily due to misconceptions about dairy fat. While dairy fats comprise the bulk of the Calories in dairy products, the *kinds* of fats in dairy products are of particular interest nutritionally. Milk is a fascinating natural food, containing approximately 400 different fatty acids, most of which are essential to good health and many of which can be found nowhere else in nature. That's why mammals thrive on it for months of life before eating solid foods.

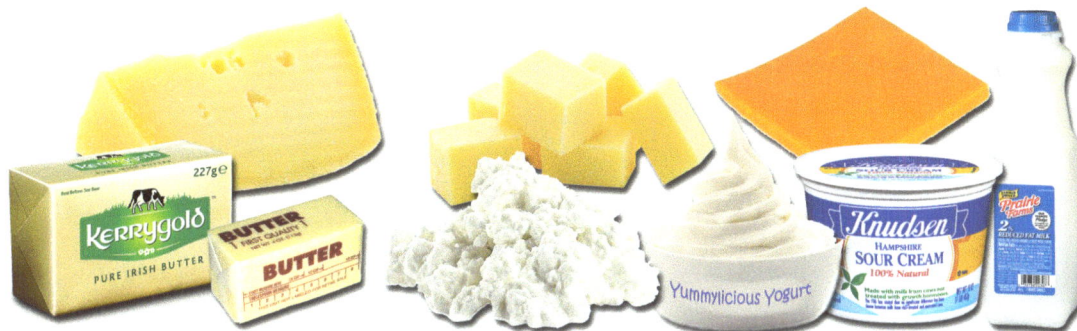

Dairy products have other substances that cause health issues in sensitive individuals. Milk contains *lactose* (milk sugar), to which about 40% of the world's adult population is intolerant due to a lack or reduced production of lactase, the enzyme necessary to break down lactose. A small percentage of people are allergic to milk protein (*casein*), or to the foods that cows eat (mostly grains and dried legumes). Grain-fed cattle are continually dosed with antibiotics and growth hormones to increase milk production, and these chemicals are passed on to you in their milk and meat. Though these health concerns are valid, nearly 60% of the world's population not only tolerates, but enjoys the benefits of dairy products in their diets. Grass-fed cows produce superior milk that is higher in omega-3s than that from grain-fed cows.

Dairy products provide immediate energy from the types of fats it possesses—notably significant amounts of short- and medium-chain fatty acids, which are burned for fuel, rather than stored as adipose tissue. In the presence of fiber, favorable intestinal bacteria ferment *butyric acid* (a short-chain fatty acid) found in butter, promoting digestive health. Dairy is perhaps the best food source of protein-bound calcium, vastly more bioavailable than ionic (unbound to protein) plant calcium sources.

Just a few years ago, consuming butterfat as found in butter, whole-fat yogurt, sour cream, and cream cheese, was considered dietary suicide. We were admonished to replace dairy fat with polyunsaturated fats, swap margarine for butter, and avoid whole-milk dairy products in favor of low- or non-fat products.

New research reveals the folly of this advice. It is the polyunsaturated omega-6 fatty acids—*not* saturated fat—that form the major fatty components of arterial plaque, yet for many years the American Heart Association and many establishment nutrition advocates emphasized consumption of polyunsaturated oils for the heart. This advice sickened or killed millions of people.

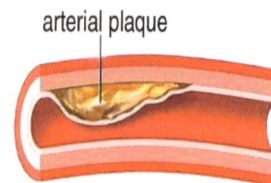

arterial plaque

The evolving wisdom recommends replacing long-chain fatty acids, in fats such as margarine and canola oil (which also contains heart-damaging *erucic* acid), with fats high in short- and medium-chain fatty acids, such as butter and tropical (coconut and palm) oils.

The table below illustrates some of the types of fats found in dairy products (percentages are *averages* from several farms).

Dairy Fat Constituents Table	
COMPONENT	PERCENTAGE
Long-Chain Fatty Acids	
Saturated Fats	70.00%
Palmitic Acid component	30.00%
Myristic Acid component	11.00%
Stearic Acid component	12.00%
Caproic Acid component	2.40%
Trans Fatty Acid component (vaccinic acid)	2.70%
Polyunsaturated Fats	2.30%
Linoleic Acid component	1.60%
α-Linolenic Acid component	.70%
Conjugated Linoleic Acid (CLA) component	1.00%
Monounsaturated Fats	25.00%
Oleic Acid component	24.00%
Short-Chain Fatty Acids	10.90%
Butyric Acid component	4.40%

Conclusion

Polyunsaturated omega-6 vegetable oils are *not found* in significant quantities in nature—man creates them mostly from heavily processing grains and seeds. Human physiology does not know how to metabolize these manufactured pseudo-foods. These foreign foodstuffs stimulate distortions in hormone and enzyme profiles that cause inflammation and lead to disease states.

Moderate dairy product and tropical oil intake improves metabolism and promotes fat loss. The human body has evolved to efficiently metabolize these fats.

Ratios of Saturated, Polyunsaturated, and Monounsaturated Fats

The typical American diet provides an imbalance of polyunsaturated over monounsaturated fats, which leads to inflammatory disease states—predominantly heart disease. Both saturated and unsaturated fat intake increases with fast-food consumption. Researchers have found that the proper ratio of the three classes of fats leads to better health.

The average American dietary intake of fats is 140–170 grams (mostly because of fast-foods)—which gravely exceeds the 30–60 grams recommended by most nutritional experts. Ideally, omega-6 to omega-3 ratios should be 1:1 in the human body, and therefore the diet. The omega-6 to omega-3 ratio in the typical industrialized diet ranges from 10:1 to 30:1, which is directly responsible for inflammatory disease states. According to research worldwide, diets that maintain a ratio of polyunsaturated to monounsaturated to saturated fats at about 2:2:1, produce the least disease.

Instructions

You will use two tables to look up foods for fat content—one for saturated and unsaturated fats (which includes both polyunsaturated and monounsaturated fractions), and the other for omega-3 fats. Refer to your Food Journal to look up the kinds of fats in your foods, so you can fill out the blank table in the Self-Assessment section.

Saturated & Unsaturated Fats Table					
FOOD	QUANTITY	TOTAL GRAMS	SATURATED GRAMS	PERCENT SATURATED	UNSATURATED GRAMS	PERCENT UNSAT.
MEATS						
Beef, heart	4 oz	3.18	1.25	39%	1.93	61%
Beef, lean ground	4 oz	11.35	5.79	51%	5.56	49%
Beef, roast	4 oz	18.75	9.56	51%	9.19	49%
Beef, sirloin	4 oz	28.00	14.28	51%	13.72	49%
Bologna, meat	4 oz	33.20	14.61	44%	18.59	56%
Chicken, dark	4 oz	7.68	2.46	32%	5.22	68%
Chicken, light	4 oz	4.50	1.49	33%	3.01	67%
Chicken, livers	4 oz	4.67	2.05	44%	2.62	56%
Franks, meat	2 wieners	20.00	8.80	44%	11.21	56%
Lamb, chops	4 oz	24.25	13.82	57%	10.43	43%
Lamb, roast leg	4 oz	15.43	8.80	57%	6.63	43%
Pork, bacon	4 oz	78.50	32.19	41%	46.32	59%

Saturated & Unsaturated Fats Table, continued					
FOOD	QUANTITY	TOTAL GRAMS	SATURATED GRAMS	PERCENT SATURATED	UNSATURATED GRAMS	PERCENT UNSAT.
Pork, chops	4 oz	22.25	9.12	41%	13.13	59%
Pork, roast	4 oz	26.00	10.66	41%	15.34	59%
Pork, sausage	4 oz	57.50	23.58	41%	33.92	59%
Pork, spareribs	4 oz	22.43	9.20	41%	13.23	59%
Turkey, dark	4 oz	9.40	2.91	31%	6.49	69%
Turkey, light	4 oz	4.43	1.37	31%	3.06	69%
Veal, cutlet	4 oz	10.30	5.25	51%	5.05	49%
GAME						
Duck	4 oz	35.50	9.10	26%	23.40	74%
Goose	4 oz	38.50	12.32	32%	26.18	68%
Pheasant	4 oz	11.75	4.00	34%	7.75	66%
Rabbit	4 oz	7.25	1.81	25%	5.44	75%
Venison	4 oz	4.50	3.11	69%	1.40	31%
DAIRY						
Buttermilk	1 cup	5.00	3.30	66%	1.70	34%
Cheese, American	1 oz	8.86	5.85	66%	3.01	34%
Cheese, Bleu	1 oz	8.40	5.32	65%	2.66	35%
Cheese, cheddar	1 oz	9.40	5.98	64%	2.93	36%
Cheese, cottage low-fat	4 oz	2.00	1.32	66%	0.68	34%
Cheese, cottage reg.	4 oz	5.00	3.30	66%	1.70	34%
Cheese, cream	1 oz	10.6	7.00	66%	3.60	34%
Cheese, Mozzarella	1 oz	4.85	3.20	66%	1.65	34%
Cheese, Muenster	1 oz	8.52	5.42	64%	2.66	36%
Cheese, Parmesan	1 oz	7.30	4.65	66%	2.29	34%
Cheese, Parmesan, dry	1 oz	3.00	1.90	63%	0.94	37%
Cream, heavy	1 oz	11.01	7.27	66%	3.74	34%
Eggs	1 large	6.00	2.70	45%	3.30	55%
Ice cream	8 oz	14.3	9.44	66%	4.86	34%
Ice milk	8 oz	5.63	3.51	62%	1.84	38%
Milk, low-fat	1 cup	4.68	2.92	66%	1.52	34%
Milk, whole	1 cup	8.15	5.38	66%	2.77	34%
Yogurt, low-fat	1 cup	3.52	2.27	64%	1.07	36%
NUTS						
Almonds, raw	2 oz	19.25	1.55	8%	16.75	92%

Saturated & Unsaturated Fats Table, continued					
FOOD	QUANTITY	TOTAL GRAMS	SATURATED GRAMS	PERCENT SATURATED	UNSATURATED GRAMS	PERCENT UNSAT.
Brazils nuts	2 oz	23.43	4.68	20%	17.33	80%
Cashews	2 oz	16.00	2.73	17%	12.33	83%
Coconut meat	2 oz	7.05	6.98	99%	0.07	1%
Peanuts	2 oz	17.53	4.03	23%	13.50	77%
Pecans	2 oz	19.23	1.54	8%	17.69	92%
Pistachios	2 oz	32.00	4.40	14%	26.00	86%
Pumpkin seeds	2 oz	16.35	3.11	19%	13.24	81%
Sunflower seeds	2 oz	17.15	2.23	13%	14.92	87%
FATS, OILS						
Butter	1 T	11.00	7.26	66%	3.74	34%
Lard	1 T	11	4.4	40.00%	6.6	60%
Margarine	1 T	11	2.09	19.00%	8.91	81%
Oil, canola	1 T	14	1	7.00%	13	93%
Oil, corn	1 T	14	1.54	11.00%	12.46	89%
Oil, olive	1 T	14	1.68	12.00%	12.32	88%
Oil, peanut	1 T	14	1.68	12.00%	12.32	88%
Oil, safflower	1 T	14	1.26	9.00%	12.74	91%
Oil, soy	1 T	14	2.38	17.00%	11.62	83%
Oil, sunflower	1 T	14	1.82	13.00%	12.18	87%
Oil, wheat germ	1 T	14	2.94	21.00%	11.06	79%
Shortening, vegetable	1 T	11	2.86	26.00%	8.14	74%

Omega-3 Fats Table	
SEAFOOD	MG/4 OZ
Bass, sea	800
Clams	274
Cod	229
Flounder	343
Haddock	229
Halibut	1486
Lobster	69
Mackerel	2171
Mussels	491
Oysters, domestic	583
Perch, freshwater	229
Red snapper	686
Salmon, pink	2514
Sardines, in oil	5829
Scallops, bay	149
scallops, sea	206
Shrimp	229
Sole	114
Swordfish	1029
Trout, freshwater	1600
Tuna, albacore	2400

Self-Assessment

Use your Food Journal on page 25 to fill out this table to analyze your fat ratios.

Fat Ratio Intake Table				
FOOD	QUANTITY	SATURATED	UNSATURATED	OMEGA-3s
TOTAL EACH TYPE, THEN ADD ALL HERE:				
DIVIDE EACH TYPE BY TOTAL FAT →	RATIO:			
MULTIPLY RATIOS BY 100 →	PERCENT:	____ %	____ %	____ %

(Fat Type / Total Fat = *Ratio*) x 100 = percentage (%)

Recall that the *ideal ratio* of unsaturated to omega-3s to saturated fats is 2:2:1. That means that unsaturated and omega-3 fats should be about the same, and you should be getting *half* (50%) of the saturated fat in your diet as the other two. This is not as easy as it seems. You may find that omega-3 supplementation will probably be necessary to approach this ratio.

HEALTH CONCEPT #4

Processed Food

Assess Your Processed Food Intake

How much processed food are you eating? Processed food has been directly linked to obesity and other disease. If the Calories from processed foods exceeds 10% of total daily calories, you may want to reconsider your choices. Ideally, a diet with no processed foods would be the most healthful, but this is probably an unrealistic expectation given mass media's "temptation marketing engine."

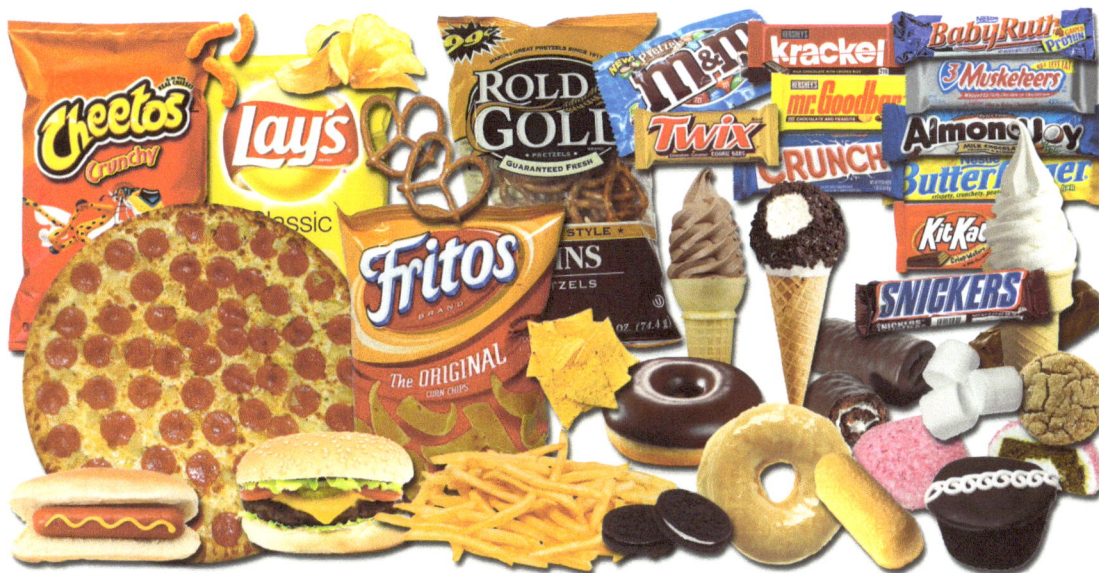

Instructions

From the table on the next pages, calculate how many calories you are consuming from processed foods. This table is just a short selection, with Calories averaged over brands, of all possible processed foods. For a more accurate assessment of your processed food intake, consult the tables at the back of this book, a nutrition manual, or the Internet for more complete Food Composition Tables that include processed, brand-name foods. A good website where you can look up foods is at:

HTTP://WWW.CALORIEKING.COM or

HTTP://NUTRITIONDATA.SELF.COM/

Calories in Common Processed Foods		
AMOUNT	**FOOD**	**CALORIES**
1 slice	Bacon	35
1 medium (3½-inch)	Bagel, white	289
1 T	Sauce, Barbecue	16
1 T	Sauce, Seafood Cocktail	60
1 T	Sauce, Tartar	35
12 oz can	Beverages, soft drinks	140
1 2-inch	Biscuit	103
1 slice	Bread, white	67
1	Bun, hamburger or hotdog	118
¹⁄₁₀ of a cake	Cake, devil's food	172
1	Cake, Hostess® cupcake	157
1	Cake, Hostess Twinkie®	150
1 2-oz	Candy bar, Snickers®	270
1 oz	Candy bar, Reese's peanut butter cup	184
1 oz	Cereal, dry breakfast	100
1 oz	"Cheesy Poofs" (Cheetos®, etc.)	159
1 drumstick	Chicken, fried, KFC®	147
1 slice	Cold Cuts, bologna	73
1	Cookies, Oreo®	49
1	Cookies, chocolate chip	51
1	Cookies, vanilla wafer	17
1 oz	Corn Nuts®	120
5	Crackers, Cheezits®	81
1	Doughnut, glazed plain	190
1	Doughnut, raised	125
1 8.5 oz can	Energy drinks (Monster®, Red Bull®, etc.)	113
1	English muffins	129

Calories in Common Processed Foods, continued		
AMOUNT	**FOOD**	**CALORIES**
1	Fish, fried sticks	40
1 small package	French fries, fast food restaurant	220
1	Frozen Dinner ("TV" type, Swanson® turkey)	540
½ can	Ham, Deviled	220
⅓ package	Hamburger Helper®	320
1 T	Jam, Jelly	67
1 T	Ketchup	18
1 T	Mayonnaise	103
1 4-inch	Pancake	54
1 cup	Pasta, regular white—any shape	197
⅙ of a 9-inch	Pie, apple	418
⅛ of a 14-inch pie	Pizza, cheese, average of all brands	300
⅛ of a 14-inch pie	Pizza, pepperoni, average of all brands	331
1 oz	Potato chips	100
1 cup	Potatoes, instant mashed	198
1 oz	Pretzels	111
1 cup	Rice, white refined, cooked	219
1 T	Salad dressing, bottled, oil-based	85
1 oz	Spam	87
1 9-inch	Tortilla, white flour	163
1 6-inch	Waffle	207
1	Wieners (all meat hot dogs/franks)	122
6 oz cup	Yogurt, sweetened fruity	110

Instructions

Fill in the table below, indicating the amounts, kinds, and Calories in the processed food you eat in one day.

	My Processed Food List	
AMOUNT	**FOOD**	**CALORIES**
	Total Processed Food Calories:	

Self-Assessment

1. In the blank below, enter the total Calories you consume in a typical day (from Health Concept #3, Your 24-Hour Food Journal).

   _____

2. Calculate the percentage of Processed Foods consumed:

   _____

   Processed Food Calories ÷ Total Food Calories = _____ x 100 = _____ % Processed Food

3. Is your processed food intake more than 10% of your total daily Calories? _____

HEALTH CONCEPT #5

Dieting Strategies

Dubious "Fad" Diets

The following fad diets have all been popular at one time or another. Short-term weight loss (not necessarily *fat* loss) can be dramatic, but the effects do not promote the kind of lifelong health that keeps dieters on them for very long. Except for Atkin's-type diets (which will still require supplementation), these fad diets are generally unsafe and ineffective for long-term fat loss and optimum health. Let's take a closer look at them....

Low-Calorie Diet (Weight Watchers, etc.)

While low-calorie diets (intake of 1000 or fewer Calories daily) do have some short-term success, they do not have long-term health effects because people cannot generally stay on them for very long. Hunger is a major factor in the ability to stick with low-calorie diets. In commercial programs such as Weight Watchers, the predominant strategy is to reduce fat intake, replacing fat Calories with carbohydrate Calories. Recall that fat contains 9 Calories per gram, vs. 4 Calories per gram for carbohydrates.

The Weight Watchers PointsPlus® system encourages (perhaps not-so-inadvertently) replacing healthful foods with sugary treats, counting the *points* rather than focusing on health. The marketing mantra, "PointsPlus values help you continue to eat the foods you like and still lose weight," is irresistible to dieters. Weight Watchers markets low-fat, high-sugar processed products to lure dieters into false confidence that they are doing the right thing by eating their products. While dining in restaurants with Weight Watchers fans, the author has observed meal companions forgo salads because of the fatty dressings, and order low-fat sugary pie for dessert, proud they've stayed within their point allowances. However, research is loud and clear on increasing sugar in the diet while lowering fats: dieters are doomed to failure, coming back to meetings week after week, abandoning the diet, going back on, and generally "yo-yo-ing" their way to misery. Weight Watchers adherents are constantly hungry because their hormone profiles are seriously distorted because of the high sugar intake. The diet industry has a $61-billion market-share and there won't be any changes to commercial diet approaches any time in the future.

Particularity in Food Selection

There are two variations of this approach to dieting. One method asserts that you must eat a certain amount of a particular food before eating your meals. For example, the Eat-

Six-Grapefruits-Per-Day diet instructs you to eat two grapefruits before each of the three meals of the day. Though grapefruit enzymes do have some modest fat-burning properties, the idea behind eating so many grapefruits is more about filling you up with low-calorie foods so you eat less of higher-calorie foods.

The second variation of this diet approach states that you can eat all you want from a narrow list of foods—for example, the Unlimited-Hard-Boiled-Eggs diet, Rice diet, and Popcorn diet. These diets are based on the faulty assumption that some particular foods are somehow "magical" in promoting weight loss. Again, this approach is more about displacing higher-calorie foods with lower-calories ones.

Both versions of this dieting strategy create nutritional imbalances which may result in health problems. For example, excessive intake of citrus fruit may cause a loss of minerals through increased urination. In some sensitive people, acidic foods may cause a rise in the body's pH. Eating unlimited amounts of protein, explained later in this section, is hard on the kidneys and may also result in mineral losses. Eating loads of rice is very *hyperglycemic* (raises blood sugar), and can cause *hyperinsulinism* (explained later), diabetes, and fat gain.

One-Food-A-Day Diet

Eating only one kind of food per day can create deficiency states, as well as unusual nutrient imbalances. Most nutrients are required on a daily basis, and don't sit and "wait around" for the synergistic partner to be introduced the next day. Protein utilization is especially sensitive to such restrictions.

Arbitrary elimination of macro-nutrients from the diet may also alter the production of enzymes necessary for their digestion. Vegans reduce production of protein-digestion enzymes; sneaking animal protein into the diet can literally make a vegan sick because of reduced ability to break down the animal protein—further confirming the belief that eating meat is wrong. Low-carbohydrate dieters oftentimes experience bloating and other digestive upsets when re-introducing starches into the diet.

Special Prepared Meals (Jenny Craig, etc.)

The success of this approach to dieting is the result of two factors. If you are paying handsomely for special prepared foods, then you are motivated to stay on the diet. Also, someone other than you has planned a reasonably good-tasting meal that is not high in Calories. However, these packaged foods are highly processed, refined, and contain preservatives and flavor enhancers. Also, a conspicuous requirement of this diet is that you must provide your own produce, low-fat dairy, and lean meats. In a healthful diet, that is mostly what you're supposed to be eating, anyway!

Eliminating Food "Villains"

There are two variations of this approach to dieting. One version is subtle and is achieved by simply eliminating something—like sweets or extra fats, such as sour cream or butter. This strategy is essentially rational and not especially unhealthful.

The second version is an extreme approach exemplified by the Pritikin-type of diet during which dieters do away with most fat-containing foods. Though proponents have enjoyed some success with cardiac patients, it should never be attempted outside a clinical setting as it does indeed create nutritional imbalances that can prove life-threatening. Eliminating fats from your diet has serious consequences, the least of which are fat-soluble vitamin and mineral assimilation problems leading to hormone and metabolic issues. Susceptibility to a particular kind of stroke (intraparenchymal hemorrhage) is also increased by eliminating fats from the diet. Eliminating fats also translates to reduced protein intake and increased starch consumption to make up the Calorie deficit. High carbohydrate diets can cause hyperinsulinism (and associated health problems) in the majority of people who adopt this diet. Those interested only in weight reduction (and not disease reversal) will do well to avoid this diet or diets similar to it, unless specifically prescribed by a health professional.

High-Protein, Low-Carbohydrate Diet (Atkin's, Ketogenic)

This diet is based on the theory that protein does not convert to adipose tissue, even in gargantuan amounts, and therefore the dieter can eat as much as is desired. A concurrent severe restriction of carbohydrates (fewer than six grams daily in stage 1 of this diet) forces the system to convert protein to immediate fuel as well as accelerate adipose catabolism through ketogenesis (production of ketones—the by-products of fat breakdown). In a healthy system, about 58% of ingested protein is converted to glucose, so immediate fuel is supplied once the metabolism adjusts to this diet.

This diet works, but may be hazardous for some individuals. The metabolic rate is generally increased, blood sugar is stabilized, blood pressure may be decreased due to water loss. There is a high satiation rate, but the diet may become barely palatable after a time. Muscle-tissue wasting, often observed with low-calorie diets, is prevented with this diet. The initial dramatic weight loss often observed with this diet is due to protein overload (resulting in increased ammonia and urate) and *ketone* accumulation, forcing the kidneys to work overtime to rid the system of these potentially damaging substances. Water loss is prominent.

Ketogenesis occurs primarily from breakdown of adipose tissue, and partially from the high-fat content inherent in the standard diet. High levels of serum ketones can cause acidosis in sensitive individuals if the metabolic buffer system (mostly handled by the kidneys) is inadequate. Ketones are disposed of through, and can be measured in the urine, breath, saliva, and sweat. Since the kidneys must bear the burden of ketone flushing almost totally in a sedentary individual, release of ketones through exercise-induced sweating and exhaled air will prevent damage to these hard-working organs.

This diet is much too high in phosphorus, therefore calcium and magnesium supplementation is absolutely essential. Bicarbonate supplementation may be wise to ameliorate the systemic acidosis of a high-protein intake. Uric acid buildup is also likely if pyridoxine (B6) is not supplemented along with B-complex, otherwise gout is a possible consequence. Because fruits are forbidden, supplements of ascorbate are also necessary.

Though fresh greens are part of the diet, fiber intake is inadequate and supplemental fiber powders may be required to prevent constipation and other intestinal problems. As the fat content may also be too high, this diet is recommended only for active people with a healthy liver. Generally, long-term use of this diet is wise only while under the care and supervision of a competent health care professional.

Water-Loading Diet

High intake of purified water (up to five quarts daily) is the basis for this "toxin and fat flushing" diet. Sodium intake is also severely restricted as part of the regimen. The theory is that most people suffer from water retention due to excessive sodium intake, so flushing the system will create a groundwork for a more healthy life-style.

Food intake for the first few weeks is very limited. Turkey, eggs, fish, and green vegetables are the main staples of the diet; red meats and dairy products are used sparingly, if at all. The daily caloric intake rarely exceeds 600–800 calories. Potassium and B-vitamin supplements are advocated to accentuate the water-flushing effects of the diet. Weight loss may be quite rapid as serum sodium levels decline and water retention subsides. Many people on this diet feel better, but others may feel worse, even terrible.

Heavy water intake combined with severe sodium restriction and potassium supplementation may pose a danger to some individuals, especially those who exercise vigorously. Mineral losses (calcium, magnesium, zinc) through perspiration and pronounced diuresis, may be high and cause deficiencies. Sodium depletion through a combination of water loading, exercise, and hot weather may bring about "water intoxication" which resembles heat exhaustion—manifested as fatigue, dizziness, muscle weakness and cramping, rapid and weak pulse, and heart palpitations leading to cardiac arrest.

Protein intake on this diet during the first week or so is inadequate, thereby promoting weight loss through muscle-tissue cannibalization. This is accelerated with heavy exercise. This diet may be dangerous for more than three or four days.

Liquid Protein Diet (Protein-Sparing)

This diet is a desperate and extreme measure to promote rapid weight loss in the extremely obese (400 pounds or more). It consists of little or no solid food, with 15–60 grams of liquid protein administered daily to prevent significant muscle-tissue breakdown. Adipose tissue is rapidly broken down, and it alone provides all of the necessary energy required by the body. Ketosis is expected and marked. Because of the obvious limitations of this reducing method, heavy supplementation of most minerals is mandatory. Supplementation with B-complex vitamins is required to properly convert fat to glucose and then to ATP energy, and to mitigate the incredible physical stress associated with this starvation technique. This reducing regimen can be very dangerous. It is never recommended without the supervision of a physician, as frequent lab tests are critical. Fatalities from cardiac arrest have been reported, even under a doctor's close watch.

Herbal Powder Diets (Herbalife, etc.)

Low-calorie weight loss programs used in conjunction with herbal powders are very popular. Most of the herbs in the formulas promote diuresis and intestinal purging (diarrhea). These effects may compromise mineral balance and create serious problems in those predisposed to kidney disease or bowl afflictions, such as colitis. Herbs can be very allergenic or even toxic when combined with prescription drugs. This diet should be undertaken with the counseling of a *qualified* health professional (not a salesperson called a "counselor").

Fruit-Loading Diet (Beverly Hills or Hollywood Diets)

This diet is based on the false and unfounded claim that certain fruits (mainly pineapple and papaya) contain enzymes that promote their digestion (they do), but don't cause weight gain because they are quickly and fully digested. Furthermore, it is claimed that other foods cause weight gain because they are *not* fully digested, and the undigested residue is stored as adipose tissue. The proponents of this diet also assert that the body will use the massive quantities of sugar for immediate energy only, and that no excess intake of carbohydrates will be stored as fat. Improper food combining is also blamed as a cause for weight gain. All of this could not be further from the truth.

Undigested foods pass out of the body as feces. All-fruit diets will promote diarrhea; sodium restriction coupled with a high potassium intake will promote further water losses from tissues. Muscle-tissue breakdown will be significant if this regimen is maintained for over a week. Calcium, magnesium, zinc, and other micro-minerals are all absent. Most fruits contain little of the B-complex vitamins, and the laxative effects of this diet will further aggravate mineral and B-complex inadequacies, eventually causing severe depletion of these nutrients. Blood sugar levels may rise and fall rapidly. Absorption of fat-soluble vitamins will be greatly reduced. As a final note, this diet is very dangerous for longer than a week, and may create more problems than it alleviates. The "research" on which it is based has not been scientifically substantiated and the written work for its promotion and application is riddled with blatantly false statements, misinformation, and negligent assertions. *Dieter, beware!*

HCG Injections (Human Chorionic Gonadotropin shots)

Injection of gonadotropic hormones had been a popular reducing strategy in the past, but has recently enjoyed a resurgence since losing favor for a few years due to some of the side-effects. A low-calorie diet is used in conjunction with the shots; the diet alone promotes weight loss, while the shots curb the appetite and keep energy levels up. Gonadotropin, a pituitary hormone, can be unsafe over extended periods. This hormone affects the pituitary directly and can cause dramatic changes in every other gland/hormone system. Some side-effects are an increase or decrease in thyroid function (changing metabolic rate), and an increase or decrease in sex hormone production, which can affect sex drive and cause aberrations in the menstrual cycle. This reducing technique must be medically supervised. As with all calorie-restricted diets, supplementation of most vitamins and minerals is recommended.

The Most Important Concept You'll Ever Learn:
Insulin, Hyperinsulinism, and Inflammation

Insulin is an important metabolic hormone and is critical to health. It serves to "push" sugar into cells, where it may be broken down into energy. Insulin also keeps the blood sugar from escalating too high with excess carbohydrate intake.

That's the good news. The bad news is that this natural metabolic response becomes distorted with chronic high-carbohydrate intake, especially of the refined and processed variety. Refined and processed grain products from wheat, rice, and corn (prevalent in junk and fast foods), excessive intake of cooked root vegetables (such as potatoes, beets, and carrots), and sugars such as glucose, sucrose, and maltose, promote *hyperglycemia*—high blood sugar. Years of high-carbohydrate intake (and resultant hyperglycemic response) cause an exaggerated insulin response called *hyperinsulinism*—a pro-inflammatory state that leads to diseases such as metabolic syndrome, type-2 diabetes, heart disease, arthritis, and cancer. Yes, all of these diseases have a common cause—it's what goes in your mouth.

Glucagon is another hormone that is also involved in blood sugar regulation. Glucagon is produced in the pancreas, in different cells from insulin. The role of glucagon is to convert glycogen— stored body starch, found mostly in the liver, but also the muscles—to glucose. Glucagon raises blood sugar by breaking down glucose (called *gluconeogenesis*) when there is no food available. When glucagon is present, "good" eicosanoids are produced, that lead to the production of beneficial prostaglandins and other hormone-like compounds.

Recent research indicates that periodic fasting (once or twice weekly) stimulates production of favorable eicosanoids.

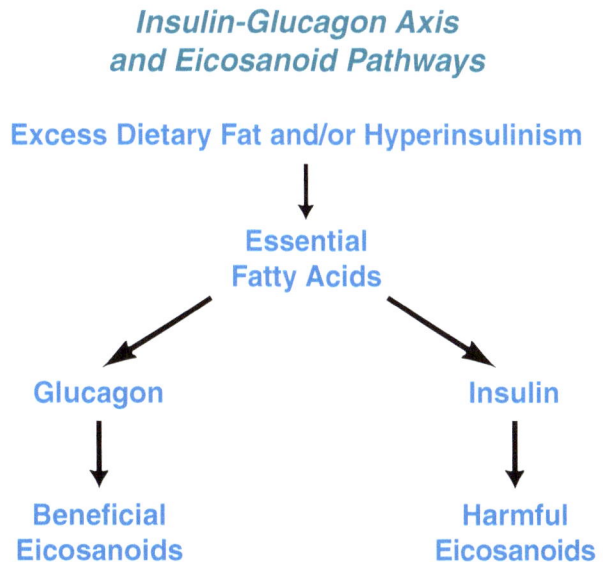

Insulin-Glucagon Axis and Eicosanoid Pathways

Excess Dietary Fat and/or Hyperinsulinism

↓

Essential Fatty Acids

↙ ↘

Glucagon **Insulin**

↓ ↓

Beneficial Eicosanoids **Harmful Eicosanoids**

Blood Sugar Table				
TIME	NORMAL	HYPOGLYCEMIC	HYPERGLYCEMIC	HYPER-HYPO*
fasting	60–100	50–70	110–130	110–120
1 hour	100–150	130–160	180–210	180–210
2 hours	90–150	80–120	220–300	220–300
3 hours	80–130	60–80	160–180	160–180
4 hours	80–100	50–70	120–140	50–70
5 hours	70–100	40–60	110–130	40–60
6 hours	60–100	40–60	110–130	40–60

* Hyper-Hypo refers to the difficult-to-manage blood glucose of the "brittle" diabetic.

Vegetable and fruit sugars such as fructose do not cause hyperinsulinism. Fructose is metabolized differently from other sugars. It does not require insulin for absorption. Instead, the liver does all the work. However, regular intake of *refined* fructose—especially that found in high-fructose corn syrup (HFCS)—raises triglycerides, causes fatty liver, and can eventually lead to non-alcoholic fatty liver disease (NAFLD) and cirrhosis. HFCS is everywhere in processed foods, some obvious such as sodas and candy bars, but much of it "hidden" in products like salad dressing; condiments; breakfast cereals; frozen, boxed, or precooked dinners; bakery goods; dairy products; fast food; snack foods; and other non-sweet products. Fructose contributes significantly to the current obesity epidemic.

Lipid (fat) synthesis is influenced by insulin levels. Increased insulin production always translates to increased serum triglycerides (blood fats). In addition, hyperinsulinism activates *hydroxymethylglutaryl coenzyme-A* (HMG CoA), an enzyme that increases cholesterol production in the liver. Increased serum lipids mean exaggerated synthesis of *arachidonic acid,* an inflammatory fatty acid.

Chronic hyperinsulinism combined with excessive dietary fat also causes insulin resistance, a condition in which cells become resistant to the sugar-clearing/storing effects of insulin, and blood sugar remains high, which can result in type-2 diabetes. Hyperglycemia in turn causes hyperlipidism and proinflammatory *eicosanoid* production. Eicosanoids are a class of polyunsaturated fatty acids that your body produces, and is also available in foods. More on this class of fats later in this section.

Insulin resistance results in the liver's *inability to suppress* glucose production from stored *glycogen* (body starch). This means that during fasting, blood glucose may go up because the liver just keeps making more from glycogen. In muscle, insulin resistance results in *impaired* glucose uptake. This lack of appropriate sensitivity towards insulin action leads to hyperglycemia (high blood sugar). Ultimately, the pancreas may fail to compensate, hyperglycemia worsens and type-2 diabetes develops.

This cascade of metabolic failures is somewhat genetically determined, but is significantly influenced by diet.

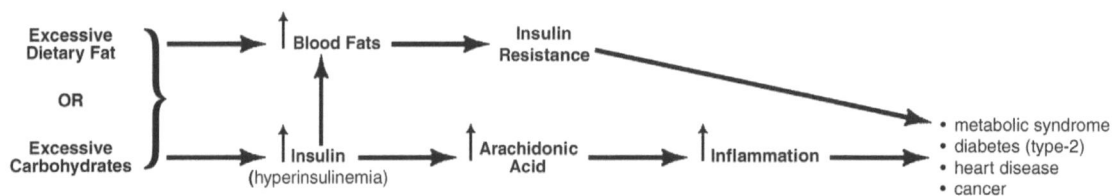

Metabolic Syndrome (sometimes called "syndrome X" or "insulin-resistance" syndrome) is a group of indicators directly related to the American refined-carbohydrate/processed-fat diet. Increased intake of refined carbohydrates (white flour, sugar, HFCS) and processed oils (polyunsaturated and hydrogenated fats) are the major culprits in this syndrome. Though type-2 diabetes and/or obesity may be present, this syndrome is *not about* either of those conditions, as the syndrome is typically expressed without type-2 diabetes or obesity. Common factors include:

- Age typically >40, but now even children can present with this syndrome

- Higher incidence in non-Caucasians

- Weight >25% normal

- Waist >40 inches—male; >35 inches—female.

- Sedentary

- Sodium/water retention

- Family history of type-2 diabetes, cardiovascular disease, coronary artery disease

- Mood shifts

- Lethargy, lack of motivation

- Tiredness

- Sleepiness

- Cravings

- Increased resting heart rate (>72)

- Fasting glucose 110–126

- Blood pressure > 140/85

- Triglycerides >150

- 2-hour blood sugar, post-75 g glucose load >140

- HDL <40—male; <50—female

- Acanthosis nigricans (a dark fungus) infections in armpits, groin, fat flaps

- LDL—APO-b marker

- Decreased leptin titer; leptin resistance

- Increased brachial artery reactivity (positive cold-pressor test suggestive)

- Increased postprandial lipids (high blood fats following a meal)

- Increased *homocysteine* levels (directly related to heart disease)

- Decreased microalbumin levels

- Increased blood clot formation (from increased thromboxane $\rightarrow$ thrombin production)

- Only 5% of Metabolic Syndrome sufferers per year develop type-2 diabetes, but 90% of diabetics have Metabolic Syndrome.

- Most obese people do not have Metabolic Syndrome, but obesity is a risk factor.

- It takes fewer calories for those with Metabolic Syndrome to gain weight.

For decades it was mostly misunderstood why carbohydrates—especially the refined varieties—caused water retention and "puffiness" in tissues of the obese. It is now mostly understood that the dramatic weight loss seen with Atkins and Paleo diets is due primarily from reduction in inflammation formerly caused by refined carbohydrates. This inflammation causes water to build-up in tissues, especially *interstitial* spaces between cells. So, if your doctor tells you it's not possible to gain a pound of weight from a four-ounce piece of cake, you know he/she doesn't understand metabolic physiology and the *hydrophilic* (water-attracting) affect of refined carbohydrates.

Glycemic Index and Glycemic Load

Not all carbohydrates are handled by the body equally. Some carbohydrates are absorbed quickly, initiating a rapid and pronounced release of insulin; other carbohydrates cause a more modest release of insulin. The absorption rate has little to do with whether carbohydrates are simple or complex.

The **Glycemic Index** is a useful modern tool in managing weight and blood glucose levels. The glycemic index indicates how much a given food raises blood sugar compared with glucose as a standard.

$$\textit{Glycemic Index} = \frac{\textbf{blood-sugar reading from } \textit{tested food}}{\textbf{blood-sugar reading from } \textit{glucose}}$$

The Glycemic Index is a ratio that compares your blood sugar levels after eating a given food, to the blood sugar level you would get from eating a specific amount of glucose. In other words, it's a scale used to compare eating a certain food to eating pure sugar.

So, a food with a glycemic index of 50 means that eating it will give you 50 percent of the blood sugar rise you'd get if you ate a specific quantity of straight glucose.

The blood-sugar-raising effects of simple and complex carbohydrates often determine how much of these macro-nutrients may be consumed without disturbing blood-glucose *homeostasis* (optimum levels of body chemistry) Foods with a high glycemic index number are absorbed readily and raise blood sugar higher than those with lower numbers, thereby stimulating overproduction of insulin that initiate pro-inflammatory processes leading to disease states. Foods with a low index number are less likely to cause wide swings in blood-sugar. In addition, fats can appreciably slow the absorption of foods with a high index number.

Glycemic Load indicates the rise in blood sugar based on *how much* of a given food is consumed. Even foods with a low glycemic index can raise blood sugar appreciably if one eats too much of it. Likewise, eating tiny amounts of high-glycemic foods will not cause a substantial rise in blood sugar. The glycemic load is much more important than the index number, but the index number is required to calculate glycemic load. Use the following table as a general guide for keeping your glycemic load as low as possible for each meal to prevent blood sugar surges and help control weight and inflammatory impact.

A low Glycemic Load is 10 or less, medium is 11–19, and 20 or greater is considered high.

Calculating Glycemic Load:

(Glycemic Index/100) x Carbohydrate Grams = Glycemic Load

Glycemic Index & Glycemic Load of Selected Foods				
FOOD	GLYCEMIC INDEX	AMOUNT	CARB GRAMS	GLYCEMIC LOAD
CONFECTIONS, SWEETS, SUGARS (HIGH-GLYCEMIC)				
Candy, Chocolate Bar, Dove Dark	23	1 oz	18	4.14
Candy, Hard Candy, Lollypop	70	6 pieces	27	18.90
Candy, Jelly Beans	78	10 pieces	10	7.80
Candy, Chocolate bar, Mars	68	3.5 oz	67	45.56
Candy, Chocolate Bar, Snickers	68	1—2-oz bar	33	22.44
Candy, Peanut M&M's	33	1.67-oz pak	28	9.24
Honey	87	1 T	17	14.79
Jam, Preserves	51	1 T	14	7.14
Sugar, Fructose	20	1 tsp	4	0.80
Sugar, Glucose	100	1 tsp	4	4.00
Sugar, Maltose	110	1 tsp	4	4.40
Sugar, Sucrose	59	1 tsp	4	2.36
				0
MUFFINS, CAKES, COOKIES (HIGH-GLYCEMIC)				0
Brownies, packaged	42	1/15 package	34	14.28
Cake, Angel food	67	1/10 cake	27	18.09
Cake, Chocolate w/chocolate frosting	41	1/10 cake	23.4	9.59
Cake, Pound, commercial	54	1/10 cake	15	8.10
Cake, Sponge	46	1/12 of cake	36	16.56
Cake, Vanilla w/vanilla frosting	42	1/8 of cake	35	14.70
Cookie, Animal Crackers	*high*	15 pieces	22	*n/a*
Cookie, Chocolate Chip (Tollhouse)	*high*	1	8	*n/a*
Cookie, Fig bar (Newton)	*high*	1	11	*n/a*

Glycemic Index & Glycemic Load of Selected Foods, continued				
FOOD	GLYCEMIC INDEX	AMOUNT	CARB GRAMS	GLYCEMIC LOAD
Cookie, Oatmeal	55	1 large	12.2	6.71
Cookie, Oreo or Hydrox	75	1	7	5.25
Cookie, Vanilla Wafer	75	1	3	2.25
Cracker, Graham	74	2 squares	10	7.40
Donut, glazed	76	1 large	38	28.88
Muffin, Blueberry	59	1 medium	23	13.57
Muffin, Bran	60	1 medium	17.2	10.32
Pastry, Cinnamon Roll	59	1 roll	17	10.03
Pie, Apple	*high*	⅙—9" pie	61	*n/a*
Pie, Boson Cream	*high*	⅛—9" pie	51	*n/a*
Pie, Pumpkin *(sugar-sweetened)*	*high*	⅙—9" pie	37	*n/a*
Sherbet	*high*	½ cup	29	*n/a*
GRAINS, BREADS, CRACKERS (HIGH-GLYCEMIC)				
Barley, cooked	25	½ cup	22	5.50
Bread, Bagel	72	1—4"	45	32.40
Bread, Corn	110	1—2" piece	13	14.30
Bread, French	95	1 slice	11	10.45
Bread, Pita, whole wheat	57	1	24	13.68
Bread, Pumpernickel	41	1 slice	12	4.92
Bread, Rye, mixed w/wheat	42	1 slice	16	6.72
Bread, Rye 100% whole	65	1 slice	12	7.80
Bread, Wheat	72	1 slice	12	8.64
Bread, White	69	1 slice	13	8.97
Buckwheat, flour	54	1 cup	33	17.82
Corn, fresh sweet (on-the-cob)	62	1 ear	21	13.02
Crackers, Melba Toast	70	4 rounds	11	7.70
Crackers, Rye Krisp	65	1 wafer	7	4.55
Croissant, Butter	67	1 medium	11	7.37
Pasta, enriched	50	1 cup	43	21.50
Pasta, whole wheat	42	1 cup	38	15.96
Popcorn	55	1 cup	11	6.05
Rice, white Basmati	52	½ cup	19	9.88
Rice, brown, cooked	66	½ cup	19	12.54

Glycemic Index & Glycemic Load of Selected Foods, continued				
FOOD	GLYCEMIC INDEX	AMOUNT	CARB GRAMS	GLYCEMIC LOAD
Rice, white, cooked	72	½ cup	25	18
Roll, Kaiser	73	1	20	14.6
Tortilla, Corn	70	1—6"	14	9.8
Tortilla,Taco Shell	68	1 medium	7	4.76
Waffle (homemade)	76	1	28	21.28
CEREALS—BREAKFAST (HIGH-GLYCEMIC)				
All Bran	51	⅓ cup	22	11.22
Bran Flakes	74	¾ cup	24	17.76
Cheerios, plain	74	1 cup	21	15.54
Corn Chex	83	1 cup	26	21.58
Corn Flakes	80	1 cup	24	19.20
Corn pops	80	1 cup	28	22.40
Grape Nuts	75	½ cup	46	34.50
Kellogg's Special K, plain	69	1 cup	22	15.18
Museli	66	1 cup	66	43.56
Oatmeal, instant dry	65	1 packet (1 oz)	19	12.35
Oatmeal, whole, prepared	58	½ cup	13	7.54
Raisin Bran	61	1 cup	45	27.45
Rice Krispies	82	1¼ cup	28	22.96
Shredded Wheat	67	1 biscuit	20	13.40
BEVERAGES (HIGH-GLYCEMIC)				
Chocolate, Hot mix	51	1 packet	23	11.73
Cola, regular carbonated	63	12-oz can	35	22.05
Gatorade powder	78	¾ scoop	15	11.70
Juice, Apple	39	1 cup	25	9.75
Juice, Cranberry Cocktail, bottled	68	1 cup	34	23.12
Juice, Grapefruit, sweetened	48	1 cup	31	14.88
Juice, Grapefruit, unsweetened	48	1 cup	24	11.52
Juice, Orange, fresh	57	1 cup	26	14.82
Juice, Orange, from concentrate	46	1 cup	29	13.34
Juice, Pineapple, canned unsweetened	46	1 cup	32	14.72
Juice, Prune	43	1 cup	45	19.35

Glycemic Index & Glycemic Load of Selected Foods, continued				
FOOD	GLYCEMIC INDEX	AMOUNT	CARB GRAMS	GLYCEMIC LOAD
Juice, Tomato	38	1 cup	10	3.80
Juice, Vegetable	43	1 cup	11	4.73
Kool-aid, sugar-sweetened	*high*	1 cup	16	*n/a*
Milk, Almond	0	1 cup	1	0
Milk, Rice	*high*	1 cup	23	*n/a*
Milk, Soy	44	1 cup	12	5.28
FRUITS (LOW- TO HIGH-GLYCEMIC)				
Apples, w/skin	39	1 medium	25	9.75
Apricot, canned in light syrup	64	1 cup	42	26.88
Apricot, fresh	32	1	5	1.60
Banana	62	1 medium	27	16.74
Cantaloupe	65	½ melon	8	5.20
Cherries, raw	23	½ cup	11	2.53
Cranberry Sauce, canned	*high*	¼ cup	27	*n/a*
Dates	50	1 date	18	9.00
Fruit Cocktail, light syrup drained	55	½ cup	18	9.90
Grapefruit	26	1 medium	21	5.46
Grapes, red or green	45	10 grapes	9	4.05
Kiwi, no skin	58	1 medium	11	6.38
Mango	51	1 cup	39	19.89
Orange	48	1 medium	16	7.68
Papaya	60	½ fruit	15	9.00
Peach	29	1 medium	10	2.90
Peaches, canned, heavy syrup	58	½ cup	22	12.76
Peaches, canned, light syrup	52	½ cup	19	9.88
Pear	34	1 medium	31	10.54
Pears, canned in pear juice	44	½ cup	16	7.04
Pineapple, raw	66	1 cup	21	13.86
Plum	25	1 medium	8	2.00
Prunes	29	½ cup	108	31.32
Raisins	64	½ cup, loose	115	73.60
Strawberries	40	1 cup	10	4.00
Watermelon	72	1 cup	7	5.04

Glycemic Index & Glycemic Load of Selected Foods, continued				
FOOD	GLYCEMIC INDEX	AMOUNT	CARB GRAMS	GLYCEMIC LOAD
LEGUMES (LOW-GLYCEMIC)				
Beans, baked	48	½ cup	35	16.80
Beans, baked Bush's brand	40	½ cup	29	11.60
Beans, Garbanzos, boiled in water	36	½ cup	20	7.20
Beans, Kidney, boiled in water	29	½ cup	20	5.80
Beans, Lima baby, boiled in water	36	½ cup	16	5.76
Beans, Lima, Large Fordhook	31	½ cup	20	6.20
Beans, Pinto, boiled in water	39	5 oz	19	7.41
Beans, Soy, dry roasted	20	½ cup	15	3.00
Lentils, boiled in water	29	½ cup	19	5.51
Peanuts	13	1 oz	4	0.52
Peanut Butter	13	1 T	3	0.39
Peas, Black-eyed	33	½ cup	21	6.93
Peas, Green frozen	48	½ cup	11	5.28
VEGETABLES, STARCHY, SUGARY (LOW- TO HIGH-GLYCEMIC)				
Beets, canned	64	½ cup	9	5.76
Beets, cooked fresh	64	½ cup	9	5.76
Carrots, cooked	46	½ cup	8	3.68
Carrots, raw	16	1 large	10	1.60
Corn, Yellow kernels	55	½ cup	17	9.35
Parsnips, cooked	97	½ cup	13	12.61
Potato, baked Russet	111	1 medium	37	41.07
Potato, Chips	60	1 oz (15 chips)	15	9.00
Potato, Sweet, baked	54	½ cup	24	12.96
Potatoes, boiled White/Red Rose	89	5 oz	27	24.03
Potatoes, dry instant flakes	88	⅓ cup	16	14.08
Potatoes, French fries, small side	65	1 pak	26	16.90
Potatoes, Hash browns	56	1 cup	45	25.20
Yam	51	½ cup	19	9.69

Glycemic Index & Glycemic Load of Selected Foods, continued

Food	Glycemic Index	Amount	Carb Grams	Glycemic Load
VEGETABLES, WATERY (LOW-GLYCEMIC)				
Asparagus	0	4 spears	4	0
Avocado		½ fruit	13	n/a
Broccoli, cooked	0	½ cup	1	0
Cabbage, cooked or Saurkraut	0	½ cup	4	0
Cabbage, raw	0	1 cup	4	0
Cauliflower	0	½ cup	3	0
Celery, raw	0	1 stalk	1	0
Corn, fresh sweet (on-the-cob)	62	1 ear	21	13.02
Green Beans	0	½ cup	3	0
Eggplant	0	½ cup	4	0
Lettuce, any variety	0	1 cup	2	0
Mushrooms, fresh raw	0	1 cup	3	0
Olives	0	1 oz	0	0
Onions, dry raw	0	½ cup	7	0
Radishes	0	10 medium	2	0
Onions, green Scallions	0	½ cup	1	0
Pumpkin, canned, unsweetened	66	½ cup	9	5.94
Spinach	0	1 cup	3	0
Squash, Summer—Patty-Pan, Zucchini	0	½ cup	3	0
Squash, Winter		½ cup	16	0
Tomato	38	1 medium	7	2.66
Tomato Paste		6-oz can	35	0
Tomato Soup	38	1 cup	34	12.92
DAIRY PRODUCTS (LOW- TO HIGH-GLYCEMIC)				
Cheese, Cottage	0	½ cup	4	0
Cheese, Hard (jack, cheddar, mozarella)	0	1 oz	0.5	0
Ice Cream	36	½ cup	17	6.12
Ice Milk, low-fat	47	½ cup	16	7.52
Milk, skim	40	1 cup	12	4.80
Milk, whole	36	1 cup	13	4.68
Pudding	44	½ cup	33	14.52
Yogurt, plain, low-fat	36	½ cup	9	3.24

Glycemic Index & Glycemic Load of Selected Foods, continued				
FOOD	GLYCEMIC INDEX	AMOUNT	CARB GRAMS	GLYCEMIC LOAD
NUTS, SEEDS (NON- TO LOW-GLYCEMIC)				
Almonds	0	1 oz (2 T)	7	0
Brazils	2	1 oz (2 T)	19	0.38
Cashews	22	1 oz (2 T)	5	1.10
Coconut Meat, shredded unsweetened	0	½ cup	4	0
Hazelnuts (Filberts)	0	1 oz (2 T)	4	0
Macadamias	0	1 oz (2 T)	4	0
Pecans	0	1 oz (2 T)	2	0
Peanuts	13	1 oz (2 T)	4	0.52
Peanut Butter	13	1 T (.5 oz)	3	0.39
Pistachios	0	1 oz (2 T)	3	0
Seeds, Pumpkin (Pepitas)	0	1 oz (2 T)	3	0
Seeds, Sesame	0	1 oz (2 T)	4	0
Seeds, Sunflower	0	1 oz (2 T)	4	0
Soybeans, dry roasted	15	1 oz (2 T)	9	1.35
Walnuts, English or Black	0	1 oz (2 T)	2	0
MEATS/PROTEIN (NON- TO LOW-GLYCEMIC)				
Beef	0	any amount	0	0
Buffalo	0	any amount	0	0
Chicken	0	any amount	0	0
Deer-Venison	0	any amount	0	0
Duck	0	any amount	0	0
Eggs	0	1	0.3	0
Elk	0	any amount	0	0
Fish	0	any amount	0	0
Fish sticks	38	1 stick	2	0.76
Ham	0	any amount	0	0
Lamb	0	any amount	0	0
Lobster	0	any amount	0	0
Ostrich	0	any amount	0	0
Pork	0	any amount	0	0
Rabbit	0	any amount	0	0
Sausage, Pork	28	1 link	3	0.84

Glycemic Index & Glycemic Load of Selected Foods, continued				
FOOD	**GLYCEMIC INDEX**	**AMOUNT**	**CARB GRAMS**	**GLYCEMIC LOAD**
Shellfish	0	any amount	0	0
Turkey	0	any amount	0	0
Veal	0	any amount	0	0
FATS (NON-GLYCEMIC)				
Butter	0	any amount	0	0
Olive Oil	0	any amount	0	0
Coconut Oil	0	any amount	0	0
Fish Oil	0	any amount	0	0
Heavy or Sour Cream	0	1 oz (2 T)	1	0
Other Vegetable Oils	0	any amount	0	0

You may wish to consult a more complete Glycemic Index list from a nutrition manual or the Internet. A good database reference for the Glycemic Index is available at the University of Sydney, Australia website at: HTTP://WWW.GLYCEMICINDEX.COM/.

Instructions

1. Enter the foods you eat for each meal in a day, and the Glycemic Index of each in the table provided on the next pages.

2. Enter the Glycemic Load for each food, adjusting for quantity. For example, if you had 4 sausage links for breakfast, you would enter 12 for the total carbohydrate grams (4 links x 3 grams of carbohydrate each) and calculate that the Glycemic Index (28)/100 x Carbohydrate Grams (12) = Glycemic Load (3.36). That is, (28/100=) = .28 x 12 =3.36

Remember This: (Glycemic Index/100) x Carbohydrate Grams = *Glycemic Load*

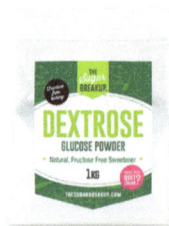

My Glycemic List				
FOOD	GLYCEMIC SCALE	AMOUNT	CARB GRAMS	GLYCEMIC LOAD
BREAKFAST				
TOTAL GLYCEMIC LOAD FOR THIS MEAL:				_____
LUNCH				
TOTAL GLYCEMIC LOAD FOR THIS MEAL:				_____
DINNER				
TOTAL GLYCEMIC LOAD FOR THIS MEAL:				_____
DESSERT				
TOTAL GLYCEMIC LOAD FOR THIS MEAL:				_____

My Glycemic List, continued				
FOOD	GLYCEMIC SCALE	AMOUNT	CARB GRAMS	GLYCEMIC LOAD
SNACKS				
TOTAL GLYCEMIC LOAD FOR THIS MEAL:				_____
TOTAL GLYCEMIC INDEX NUMBERS:				_____
AVERAGE GLYCEMIC INDEX NUMBER:				_____

Glycemic Load Scale	
SCALE	GLYCEMIC LOAD
Low	≤ 10
Medium	11–19
High	≥ 20

Self-Assessment

1. In the table you filled out above, sum up the Glycemic Index totals of all the carbohydrate sources from foods you eat in a day. Average them in the cell below the totals. *Tip:* To *average* a list of numbers, simply add all the entries, then divide by the number of entries. What is the *average* Glycemic Index of the food you ate in a day?

   _____

2. In the same table you filled out above, calculate the Glycemic Load of all the carbohydrate sources from food you eat in one meal. Add the total at the end of each meal section. *Tip:* When adding glycemic load numbers, *do not average* them. Glycemic load is *cumulative!*

3. What is your total glycemic load for breakfast? _____

4. What is your total glycemic load for lunch? _____

5. What is your total glycemic load for dinner? _____

6. What is your total glycemic load for dessert? _____

7. What is your total glycemic load for snacks? _____

8. Total the glycemic loads for all meals and snacks for the day: _____

9. Is this load typical of your daily diet? _____

10. If you are attempting to lose weight, do you think there is room for improvement?
    _____

11. Do you think you might be at risk for Metabolic Syndrome or even Type-2 Diabetes?
    _____

12. Have you followed up on blood tests to determine your blood sugar, triglyceride, and cholesterol values?
    _____

HEALTH CONCEPT #6

Energy Expenditure
During Daily Activities

How to Calculate Your BMR (Basal Metabolic Rate)

It is possible to assess how much energy you expend in a given period (and therefore how much energy you need to stay in body-weight equilibrium) using tables and calculations. You will use a *General* and a *Precise* method, and compare the results.

METHOD 1: A General Calculation involves three parameters:

- Basal Metabolic Rate (BMR)
- Metabolism/Digestion Expenditure
- Activity Level (Muscular Work)

1. The **Basal Metabolic Rate (BMR)** is the resting rate at which living systems use oxygen, required to burn food, converting matter to energy. Though oxygen consumption is best measured in a controlled laboratory environment, a simple calculation will provide a general determination:

BMR Calculation

Female   Body weight in kg x 0.9 _____

Male   Body weight in kg x 1.0 _____

= kg/hour x 24 hours = total required Calories at BMR: _____

Most people experience a 2%-per-decade drop in BMR after maturity (age 20), so factor that in if you are older than 20 years:

- If you are in your thirties, subtract 2% _____ from your Total Calories Required at BMR: _____

- If you are in your forties, subtract 4% _____ from your Total Calories Required at BMR: _____

- If you are in your fifties, subtract 6% _____ from your Total Calories Required at BMR: _____

- If you are in your sixties, subtract 8% _____ from your Total Calories Required at BMR: _____

- If you are in your seventies, subtract 10% _____ from your Total Calories Required at BMR: _____

- If you are in your eighties, subtract 12% _____ from your Total Calories Required at BMR: _____

- If you've made it into your nineties, *party on!* Nothing you change at this point is likely to make much of a difference....

2. The Cost of Food Digestion and Metabolism requires about 10% of total Caloric intake:

    Total Calories: _____ x 10%: _____ = _____

3. Activity Level (Muscular Work Performed) influences how much more energy (as a percentage of BMR) is required by a living system to maintain body weight (attain equilibrium).

Added Expenditure (% of BMR)

- Sedentary   20% _____
- Light activity   30% _____
- Moderate activity 40% _____
- Heavy activity   50% _____

Total Calculations from **1.** + **2.** + **3.** =
Total Daily Calories Required for You to Maintain Current Weight: _____

METHOD 2: Precise Energy Requirement Calculation

A more sophisticated—and more accurate—calculation for energy requirements vs. expenditure is possible using tables and charts.

Parameters

- Basal Metabolic Rate (BMR)

- Activity Level (Muscular Work)
- Metabolism/Digestion Expenditure

1. Determine Surface Area

a. Using the Surface Area Determination graph on the next page, draw a straight line from your height (right column) to your weight (left column); the crossing point shows your surface area in M². Write this number below:

_____

(For example, a person 5'8" weighing 150 lbs. has a surface area of 1.8 M².)

b. Consult the ***BMR Table*** on page 102–103 to find your age and sex, and multiply the *calorie factor* by the surface area determined in step **1a**. Write this number below:

Calorie Factor _____ x Surface Area _____ = _____ .

Surface Area Determination

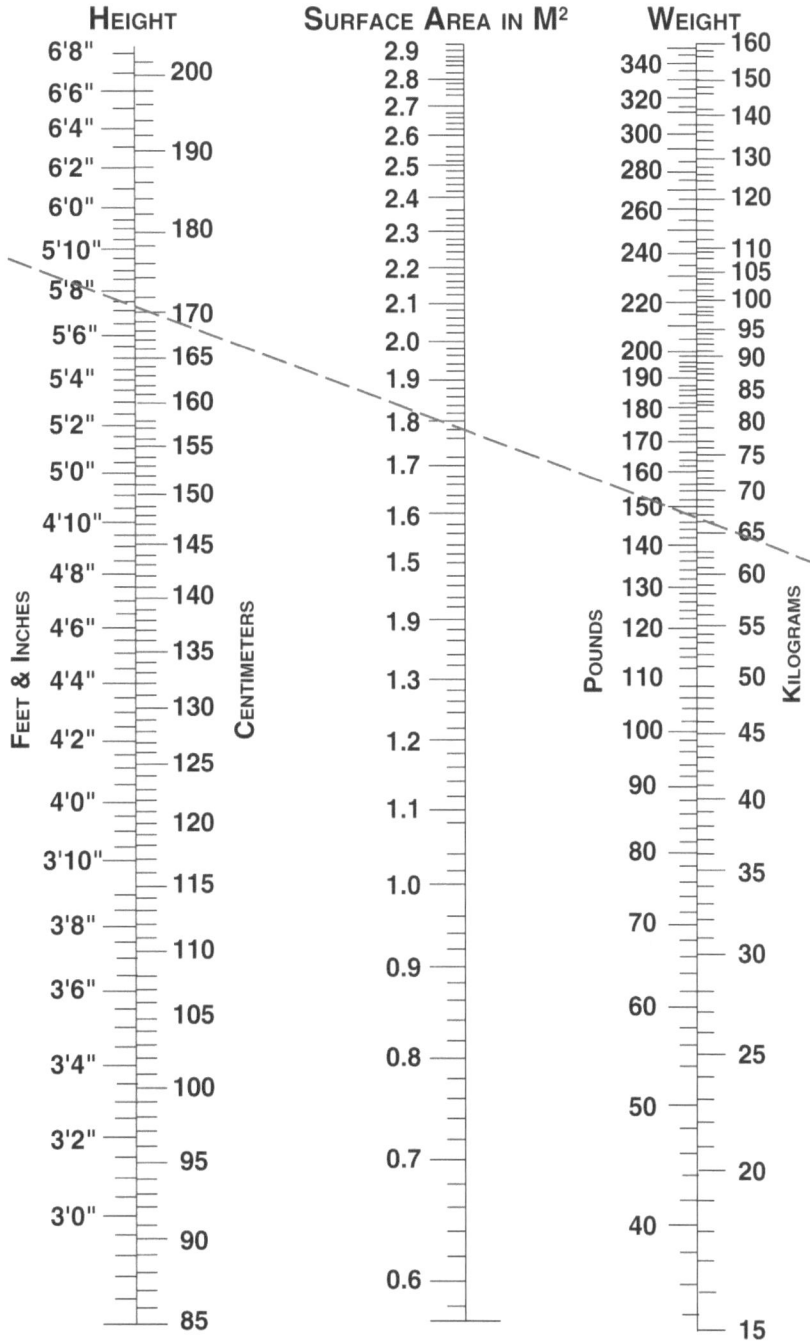

HEIGHT

6'8"	200
6'6"	
6'4"	190
6'2"	
6'0"	180
5'10"	
5'8"	170
5'6"	165
5'4"	160
5'2"	155
5'0"	150
4'10"	145
4'8"	140
4'6"	135
4'4"	130
4'2"	125
4'0"	120
3'10"	115
3'8"	110
3'6"	105
3'4"	100
3'2"	95
3'0"	90
	85

FEET & INCHES — CENTIMETERS

SURFACE AREA IN M^2

2.9
2.8
2.7
2.6
2.5
2.4
2.3
2.2
2.1
2.0
1.9
1.8
1.7
1.6
1.5
1.9
1.3
1.2
1.1
1.0
0.9
0.8
0.7
0.6

WEIGHT

340	160
320	150
300	140
280	130
260	120
240	110 / 105
220	100
200	95
190	90
180	85
170	80
160	75
150	70
140	65
130	60
120	55
110	50
100	45
90	40
80	35
70	30
60	25
50	
40	20
	15

POUNDS — KILOGRAMS

BMR Table		
AGE	MALE	FEMALE
	(KCAL/M^2/HR)	
3	60.1	54.5
4	57.9	53.9
5	56.3	53.0
6	54.0	51.2
7	52.3	49.7
8	50.8	48.0
9	49.5	46.2
10	47.7	44.9
11	46.5	43.5
12	45.3	42.0
13	44.5	40.5
14	43.8	39.2
15	42.9	38.3
16	42.0	37.2
17	41.5	36.4
18	40.8	35.8
19	40.5	35.4
20	39.9	35.3
21	39.5	35.2
22	39.2	35.2
23	39.0	35.2
24	38.7	35.1
25	38.4	35.1
26	38.2	35.0
27	38.0	35.0
28	37.8	35.0
29	37.7	35.0
30	37.6	35.0
31	37.4	35.0
32	37.2	34.9
33	37.1	34.9
34	37.0	34.9
35	36.9	34.8
36	36.8	34.7
37	36.7	34.6
38	36.7	34.5
39	36.6	34.4

BMR Table		
AGE	MALE	FEMALE
	(KCAL/M²/HR)	
40–44	36.4	34.1
45–49	36.2	33.8
50–54	35.8	33.1
55–59	35.1	32.8
60–64	34.5	32.0
70–74	32.7	31.1
75	31.8	30.9

c. Multiply the product in step **2b** by 24 (hours in a day) to determine daily BMR requirements. Write this number below:

_____ x 24 hours = _____

2. Determine Muscle Activity

a. Using the Activity Table, keep a 24-Hour Activity Journal for a typical day and record the minutes spent at each activity level in the 24-Hour Activity Level Table. Account for all 1,440 minutes in a 24-hour period.

Activity Table	
LEVEL	ACTIVITY
1	lying around, sleeping, relaxing
2	standing, sitting, reading, sewing, writing, watching TV, drawing, computing, eating, etc.
3	walking down stairs
4	very light activity: driving, slow walking on level ground
5	light activity: light housework, sweeping, moderately fast walking, carrying groceries
6	walking up stairs
7	moderate activity: fast walking, dancing, casual bicycling
8	heavy activity: fast dancing, speed walking, fast uphill walking
9	vigorous exercise: running, tennis, performance dancing, volleyball, high-intensity activity—up to 60 seconds per cycle
10	severe exercise: rowing, racing, boxing, wrestling, jumping rope, high-intensity activity—up to two minutes per cycle

b. Add the minutes spent at each energy level in appropriate columns of the 24-Hour Activity Level Table.

ACTIVITY	ACTIVITY LEVEL									
	1	2	3	4	5	6	7	8	9	10

24-Hour Activity Level Table

c. Add all the minutes spent in each activity from your 24-Hour Activity Level Table and transfer the totals to the Energy Expenditure Table. Account for all 1,440 minutes in a 24-hour period.

Energy Expenditure Table

ENERGY LEVEL	TOTAL MINUTES	CALCULATION (X KCAL/KG/MIN)	TOTAL ENERGY EXPENDED (KCAL/KG)
1		x 0.00 =	
2		x 0.01 =	
3		x 0.01 =	
4		x 0.02 =	
5		x 0.03 =	
6		x 0.04 =	
7		x 0.04 =	
8		x 0.07 =	
9		x 0.11 =	
10		x 0.14 =	
		TOTALS:	_____

3. Calculate Calorie Expenditure for Digestion and Metabolism

a. Refer to your 24-Hour Food Journal in under "Health Concept #2—Calories from Macro-Nutrients" on page 25, accounting for all calories consumed.

b. Multiply the total caloric intake from the 24-Hour Food Journal by 10%. Write this number below:

Total Calories _____ x 10% = _____

4. **Total Energy Expenditure**

   a. Add all the figures from the *Totals* in the three previous *numbered* steps. Total the calculations below:

   1. _____ + **2.** _____ + **3.** _____ = _____

   This is your total energy expenditure/requirement for one day at your current weight.

   > Many obese people find that their calculated Caloric requirements with these methods seem excessive, that they never consume this number of Calories even when tracking and measuring all foods, accounting for every Calorie ingested. Maintaining a heavy weight while eating very little, is known to occur for life-long dieters, in which metabolic rate has been greatly reduced by prolonged restriction. Extended very–low-calorie diets will backfire over the long-run because metabolic rate declines to meet demand. The diet industry capitalizes on this result. But, in such cases, only exercise can reverse this unfortunate outcome.

5. Compare your daily energy expenditure from both methods of calculation. Write the results below:

   General Calculation: _____ **Precise Calculation:** _____

   Do these figures agree? _____

   (They might not; this is just to understand how *different systems of measurement* can produce different results. Science is like that, sometimes....).

HEALTH CONCEPT #7

Exercise for Weight Control

When it comes to weight loss, diet alone rarely accomplishes satisfactory results in the long-term. In fact, reducing Calories for an extended period (longer than 10 days) will result in a reduced metabolism. This means your body adapts to a "starvation signal" so that it cuts back its energy expenditure to meet the reduced Caloric intake. Not what you want!

When using a sensible dieting strategy in conjunction with exercise, your goal is not just to lose weight, but to specifically lose body fat. In fact, many reduced-Calorie diets and exercise programs promote water and muscle tissue loss. The percentage of body fat may still be high, even though the scale reflects weight loss. The goal of a dieter should be to increase muscle while burning fat. Muscle requires more energy to maintain during rest than fat, increasing metabolism. Fat also takes up more volume than muscle. Numbers on the scale may not change much (unless the dieter is morbidly obese), but body measurements diminish as lean muscle increases. There is a specific kind of exercise that can prevent muscle tissue loss (and build more muscle), while accelerating fat loss... and it isn't "cardio"!

As always, consult with a qualified medical practitioner or fitness professional before engaging in an exercise program, especially if you are currently not fit.

Hazards of Endurance and "Cardio" Training

We humans have evolved to exert ourselves in intense bursts of activity—such as in chasing food-on-the-hoof or escaping predators. However, endurance pursuit of prey was sometimes necessary, as it caused most prey animals to overheat and collapse (they do not sweat—they pant), whereas humans *do sweat* and are able to stay cool during extended activity. But generally, endurance activity was not the usual activity in our pre-agrarian past. It is only with the advent of civilization and permanent settlements that humans had begun engaging in endurance activity—mostly in the form of competition and sport.

In modern times, though "cardio" workouts have become the gold-standard in fitness, it takes a considerable toll on human health. Many athletes—most of them runner and football players—have died of sudden cardiac arrest (SCD) either during or immediately after prolonged exertion. One of the first recorded athlete deaths was Pheidippides of Athens, a marathon-runner, who died of "exhaustion" in 490 BC. More recently, the runner Jim Fixx died at age 52 during his daily run (he did have occluded arteries), Miami Dolphins linebacker Larry Gordon (only 28 years old) died of SCD after a game, Chuck Hughes of the Detroit Lions (also 28) died of sudden cardiac arrest in-game, and Damian

Nash of the Denver Broncos died of cardiac arrest at age 24, to name just a few. Though influencing factors such as pre-existing cardiac valve, cardiomyopathy (heart muscle abnormalities), high blood-pressure, and heat-related conditions must be taken into account, the predominate cause of sudden cardiac death in young athletes is that they have never taught their hearts to *recover*. It is interesting to note, that in researching athletes who died of sudden cardiac death, that baseball player deaths of SCD were found to be rare. It is possible that heart recovery is a feature of the stop-and-start nature of the sport, so cardiac recovery strength is built into the game. The evidence is overwhelming that endurance activity is detrimental to health. Recent research verifies that this kind of activity causes unexpected stress reactions within the body. It increases metabolites and free-radicals (loose, charged particles that wreck havoc within cells) that destroy muscle tissue, including that of the heart—the opposite of what "cardio" enthusiasts want. Autopsies of marathon runners reveal smaller hearts than average, as muscle tissue is reduced to make the body more efficient for extraordinary demand. While natural testosterone and growth-hormone levels plummet, cortisol and free-radicals surge, promoting easy weight gain and accelerated aging. Joint degeneration is an expected result of endurance exercise. Luckily, the age of "cardio" is about to end, in favor of more natural and beneficial high intensity interval training.

Exercise Physiology and Benefits of High-Intensity Interval Training (HIIT)

During the first minute or two of exercise, your body burns ATP (adenosine triphosphate) for energy. (Your muscles turn glycogen into ATP energy, which is limited.) This aerobic respiration lasts for 15 to 20 minutes. To continue activities, the ATP expended has to be replaced. With high-intensity activity, ATP can't be generated with oxygen as fast as you are using it, so your muscles start to become ATP depleted. That's the point at which your anaerobic energy system kicks in. This is also known as crossing your aerobic threshold, or "hitting the wall" in runner-speak. When your anaerobic system is engaged, you are training your high-energy output system to add more energy to your "exercise furnace."

Extended endurance exercise depletes blood sugar, then depletes glycogen in muscles and the liver. Then your system resorts to breaking down proteins—muscle—for fuel. The longer this goes on, the more muscle tissue gets used for immediate fuel. This is a normal consequence of "cardio" endurance exercise, hence athletes' advice to eat lots of protein after exercise to repair damaged and lost muscle tissue.

When you stop exercising after depleting glycogen, your body shifts to a new phase and will automatically burn fat to replace the carbohydrates you just used up. This "after burn" taps the fat in storage. After a few months of high-intensity interval training, your body stops storing fat because it simply doesn't need it.

Exceeding your aerobic limit and crossing over into your "supra-aerobic zone" burns fat. By shedding the "cardio" aerobics dogma and persuading your body into its supra-aerobic zone, you'll restore native health benefits: a strong heart that knows how to rest and recover, powerful lungs, strong muscles, youthful features, no excess fat, and a longer life.

Interval training involves short bursts of intense effort. For the obese, the benefits of this kind of exercise cannot be underestimated. Since blood sugar problems and insulin-resistance are often prominent features of obesity, interval training greatly assists in regulating blood sugar and insulin sensitivity. Interval training specifically burns blood sugar, not fat. This may sound counter-intuitive if your goal is to lose weight. Also, when obese people exercise, their sheer bulk burns more Calories for the same amount of effort than a thinner person will experience. Gravity may seem like the enemy for an obese person, but they'll benefit dramatically from vigorous physical effort and lose weight faster. This is incentive enough to keep doing it!

Burning up most of your blood-sugar and glycogen stores for a short, intense duration avoids muscle breakdown for fuel, and taps the fat stores to regulate blood sugar and replace glycogen once you stop exercising. Your body enjoys a supra-aerobic state, after which it enters an anaerobic state to break down fat to replace the glycogen you burned during exertion. Most of the weight loss occurs *after* exercise, not during it. After high-intensity exercise, the body burns an even higher percentage of energy as fat (60%) while resting.

Exercise Intensity vs. Macro-Nutrients Burned			
ACTIVITY LEVEL	NUTRIENTS USED FOR IMMEDIATE FUEL		
	PROTEIN	CARBS	FAT
Low Intensity	5–8%	70%	15%
Moderate Intensity	2–5%	40%	55%
High Intensity	2%	95%	3.00%
Resting after HIIT	1–5%	35%	60%

The metabolism increases and sustains at a higher rate for about 24–48 hours after exercising stops. It is possible to increase your metabolism by several times its resting rate with regular interval exercise. As if this were not enough, interval training greatly enhances your cardiac and pulmonary reserve. Current research indicates that those with the most "lung power" enjoy longer and healthier lives. Pulmonary reserve is directly correlated to longevity.

Assessing Your Fitness Level

Before you begin or change your exercise routine, you need to evaluate your fitness level and cardiac strength.

Instructions

Formula for Calculating Maximum Heart Rate

210 – (½ age) – (5% of body weight) –4 (if male) or –0 (if female)

So, if you are a 20-year-old male and weigh 150 pounds...

210 minus half your age (10) = 200

minus 5% of body weight (150 x 5%) = 7.5

= 200–7.5 = 192.5

–4 if male = 188.5...this is your *maximum* heart rate

You'll need to exercise at 70–85% maximum heart rate to achieve fitness.

188.5 x 70% (rounded to nearest whole number) = 132

188.5 x 85% (rounded to nearest whole number) = 160

That would be 132–160 bpm (beats per minute) for a 150–pound 20-year-old male.

Self-Assessment

1. Calculate your own maximum heart rate below. (red type indicates calculations for a hypothetical 150–lb 20-year-old male)

   a. Your age: _____ (20)

   b. Half your age: _____ (10)

   c. Subtract answer in **1b** from 210: _____ (200)

   d. Your weight: _____ (150)

   e. 5% of your weight: _____ (7.5)

   f. Subtract answer in **1e** from answer in **1c**: _____ (192.5)

   g. If male, subtract 4 from answer in **1f**: _____ (188.5)
   This is your *maximum* heart rate.

2. Calculate your "exercise zone" on the next page.

a. Your maximum heart rate times 70%
(round to nearest whole number): _____ (131.95 → 132)

b. Your maximum heart rate times 85%
(round to nearest whole number): _____ (160.225 → 160)

c. Your exercise zone range is: _____ (132–160)

Finding Your Recovery Heart Rate

Your recovery heart rate—how fast your heart resumes the resting rate after intense exercise—is the best tool you have to find out if you're exercising enough, or are out of shape. If your heart does not slow down at least 30 beats in the *first minute* after stopping exercise at your zone level (70–85% of calculated maximum heart rate), you are in poor shape and at increased risk for a heart attack.

Fitness is also related to resting heart rate. Though the "average" resting heart rate is 72, it will usually be in the mid to lower 60s in a fit person. It is not unusual for an elite athlete to have a resting heart rate in the mid-50s.

Instructions

- Engage in any strenuous activity that will get your heart rate up to 70–85% of your calculated maximum rate. Use your legs predominantly.

- Measure your heart rate.

- Keep going at that pace for another minute.

- Then start a cool-down period in which you slow down to "coasting" speed. Do that for 2 minutes, then stop completely.

- Now measure your heart rate exactly 60 seconds after you stop. That's your *recovery heart rate*. Write it down here: _____ bpm

Self-Assessment

1. Calculate your exercise and recovery heart rates below.

    a. Heart rate in exercise zone for 1–2 minutes: _____

    b. Heart rate after 2-minute "coasting" cool-down and stopping: _____

    c. Heart rate after 60 seconds (1 minute) from stopping: _____

2. Calculate your recovery heart rate on the following page.

a. Heart rate in answer **1a**: _____

b. Subtract answer in **1c** from answer **2a** above: _____

Are you fit, or do you need some improvement?

Interval Training Routines

Your goal is to create an "oxygen debt" as described earlier. You must exercise at an intensity you can't sustain for more than a short period—just a few seconds to minutes. You need to demand from your lungs more oxygen than they can deliver.

How do you know if you're creating an oxygen deficit? Look at your heart rate monitor (or take your carotid or radial pulse). Always monitor your heart rate while you're engaged in interval training. When you finish an exertion period and go into a recovery period, your heart rate should *go up a few points* immediately after you slow down. If you do this successfully, you will feel yourself begin to "puff and pant."

Cardio will never work for you as well as HIIT (High Intensity Interval Training). Burning fat while exercising signals your body that it *needs* the fat, so it becomes adept at *storing* it! By creating an oxygen deficit after each interval, you are constructing a body that builds muscle and burns fat…later. If you burn glycogen and sugar (converted to ATP) *while* you exercise, your body will burn fat *after* the workout to restore its fuel levels in your muscle tissue. Doing this repeatedly, your body becomes accustomed to burning fat after each workout. The best part is, interval training isn't about duration—the ideal routine is only 10–20 minutes long!

Instructions

Though interval training uses short durations of exertion interspersed with resting periods (recovery), the most prominent feature is not that it's a modest time investment, but that as weeks progress the intensity of the exercise goes up. You can only achieve supreme fitness when *intensity continually increases.*

Study the chart on the next page. Choose a high-intensity exercise that will leave you winded after 1–2 minutes. Treadmill jogging, sprinting, swimming, bicycling, squat/thrusts, dancing, rowing, running upstairs or uphill, and jumping rope are all good ways to create an oxygen debt that burns fat. *Do not* use weights for high-intensity interval training—it can damage joints and muscles.

Sample Interval Training Routine

WARM UP	SET 1		SET 2		SET 3		SET 4		SET 5	
Minutes	Exertion	Recovery	Exertion	Recovery	Exertion	Recovery	Exertion	Recovery	Exertion	Recovery
1 minute	1 minute	2 minutes	1 minute	2 minutes	1 minute	2 minutes	1 minute	2 minutes	1 minute	2 minutes

UNFIT LEVEL Interval Training Routine

WARM UP	SET 1		SET 2		SET 3		SET 4		SET 5	
Minutes	Exertion	Recovery	Exertion	Recovery	Exertion	Recovery	Exertion	Recovery	Exertion	Recovery
1 minute	1 minute	Reach your resting HR	1 minute	Reach your resting HR	1 minute	Reach your resting HR	1 minute	Reach your resting HR	1 minute	Reach your resting HR

Sample Interval Training Regimen for GENERALLY FIT Persons

(R2, R3, etc, refers to *resistance* level)

WEEKS	WARM UP	SET 1		SET 2		SET 3		SET 4		SET 5	
	Exertion	Exertion	Recovery	Exertion	Recovery	Exertion	Recovery	Exertion	Recovery	Exertion	Recovery
1 & 2	6 mins R2	10 mins	6 mins								
3 & 4	5 mins R3	8 mins	4 mins	8 mins	4 mins						
5 & 6	5 mins R4	6 mins	3 mins	6 mins	3 mins	6 mins	3 mins				
7 & 8	4 mins R4	4 mins	2 mins	4 mins R5	2 mins	3 mins	2 mins				
8 & 10	4 mins R4	3 mins	2 mins	3 mins R5	2 mins	2 mins R6	2 mins				
11 & 12	4 mins R4	3 mins	2 mins	3 mins R5	2 mins	2 mins R6	2 mins	1 mins R7	2 mins		
13 & 14	3 mins R5	2 mins	2 mins	90 secs R6	2 mins	1 mins R7	2 mins	1 mins R8	2 mins		
15 & 16	3 mins R5	2 mins	2 mins	90 secs R6	2 mins	1 mins R7	2 mins	40 secs R8	2 mins	30 secs R9	2 mins
17 & 18	2 mins R5	2 mins	2 mins	90 secs R6	2 mins	1 mins R7	2 mins	40 secs R8	2 mins	30 secs R9	2 mins
19 & 20	1 mins R5	2 mins	2 mins	90 secs R6	2 mins	1 mins R7	2 mins	40 secs R8	2 mins	30 secs R9	2 mins

HEALTH CONCEPT #8

Micro-Nutrients:
Vitamins, Minerals, and Enzymes

Enzymes are primarily composed of proteins. Vitamins and minerals also comprise enzymes. Vitamins are considered enzyme *precursors* (or co-enzymes), and are essential to the chemistry of life.

Familiar examples of co-enzymes from the Citric Acid Cycle (Kreb's cycle) include NAD—nicotinamide adenine dinucleotide—integrating niacin (vitamin B3); FAD—flavin adenine dinucleotide, which incorporates riboflavin (vitamin B2); and pantothenic acid (B5) in α-ketoglutarate and pyruvate dehydrogenases.

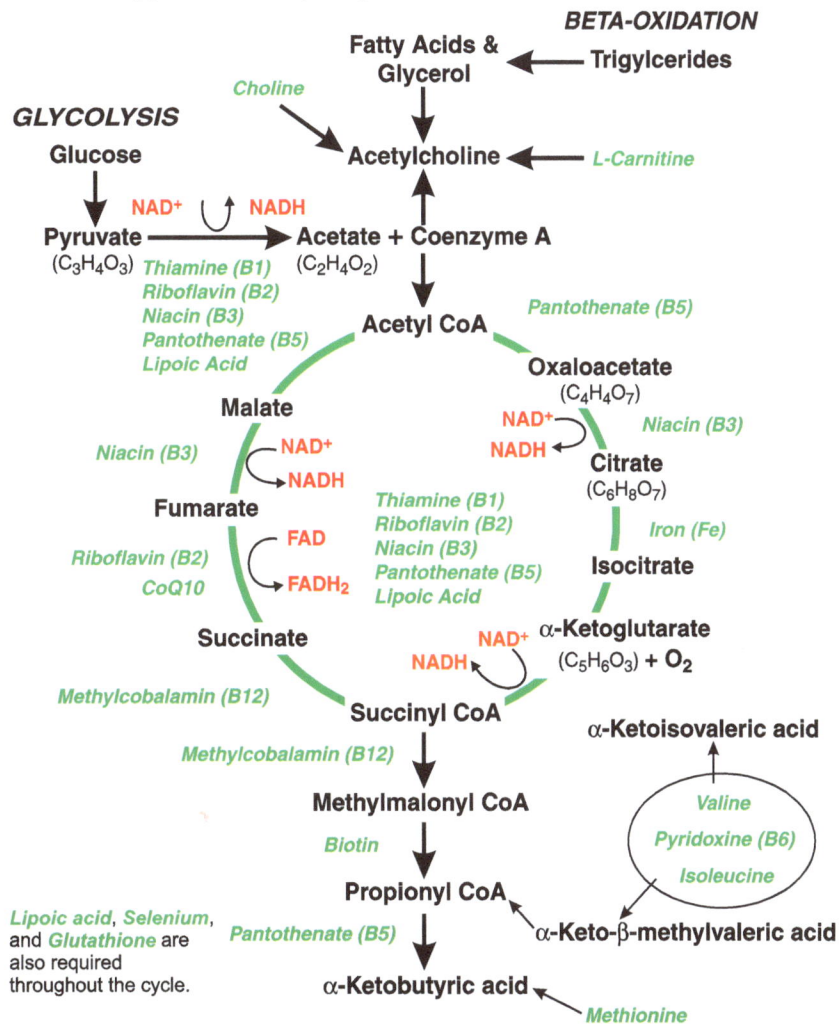

Minerals are also incorporated into enzyme systems. Iron and zinc are crucial in many enzymes; selenium is essential to production of *glutathione peroxidase,* an enzyme that protects cells from oxidative damage. Your body produces and uses thousands of enzymes—all dependent on vitamins and minerals working on a protein scaffold.

Nutrient Chirality (Polarity)

Molecules possess a property called *chirality* (ky-RAHL-i-tee), indicating its left- or right-handedness. Left-handed molecules rotate plane-polarized light (in which all light waves vibrate in the same plane) to the left (designated as *levo*), and right-handed molecules rotate plane-polarized light to the right (designated as *dextro*). The polarity affects how the charged end responds to chemical reactions. In nutrition, this property is critical to a nutrient's *bioavailability,* or the degree with which it can react with other chemicals in the body.

- Sugars are right-handed (dextro-rotatory), and are indicated by adding the letter "d" to chemical names, as in d-mannose, d-glucose, and d-ribose.

- In biologically active proteins, amino acids are left-handed (levo-rotatory), designated with the letter "l" as in l-phenylalanine, l-tryptophan, and l-lysine. (The "d"-form of amino acids exist in some bacteria and antibiotics, and in food supplements.)

- The chirality of natural vitamins is always right-handed, signified by "d" in vitamin naming conventions. Examples are d-alpha tocopherol (the alpha fraction of vitamin E) and d-ascorbate (vitamin C).

- Synthetic vitamins are left-handed, and are usually listed on food labels without the "l" designation. (This labeling deception makes them difficult to differentiate from natural forms without some education.)

- Vitamin forms with the "d-l" prefix indicate a neutral, non-reactive nutrient. The "d-l" form of vitamin E is frequently found in processed foods as a mild anti-oxidant (sprayed on breakfast cereals), cheap vitamin supplements, and lotions, indicating that the natural "d" form has been removed and replaced with a form featuring little to no bioavailability. Synthetic vitamins are several times less biologically active than natural vitamins, rendering processed food far less nutritious than its natural cousin.

Many people require or desire some vitamin supplementation as nutritional "insurance." Start with a good (not a—likely synthetic—supermarket brand) multi-vitamin, and work from there. Consult a nutritionist or vitamin-friendly doctor. Blood tests and nutritional questionnaires can help root out vitamin deficiencies. For more in-depth information on the use of vitamins and minerals, consult *Nutritional Self-Defense: Better Health in a Polluted, Over-Processed, and Stressful World* by the author.

Enzymes

Food enzymes, available only in fresh produce and raw foods, are necessary to replace and augment enzymes manufactured within the body. Without enzymes, biological processes slow or even cease, resulting in disease states and eventually death. Food enzymes are destroyed by heat, drying, prolonged exposure to light or air, preservatives, and processing. The longer fresh produce lays around, the less enzymes it contains. Processed foods contain *no natural enzymes,* and are sometimes referred to by nutritionists as "dead food."

Some people add home-grown sprouts to their diet to help supplement this valuable nutritional resource. Sprouts provide an amazing array of food enzymes and vitamins. Released from their seed chambers with just the addition of water in a jar, sprouts surrender all their nutrition before the plant uses it for its own growth. Sprouting has become one of the nation's favorite hobbies.

Preparing Foods

Produce

While most of a healthful diet consists of raw, fresh produce, there are times when cooking food is advantageous. The carotenoids (pro-vitamin A) in carrots, beets, peas, green string beans, broccoli, spinach, and other green vegetables are only about 10% bioavailable in uncooked foods. Cooking these foods fully releases some of these fat-soluble vitamins (but at the same time destroys heat-labile water-soluble vitamins such as the B vitamins and vitamin C). In addition, certain natural chemicals may be reduced with cooking. For example, *oxalic acid,* which binds to calcium in the gut making it unavailable for absorption, is reduced with cooking. Raw members of the cabbage family such as broccoli, cabbage, and Brussels sprouts, contain *glucosinolates,* which inhibit the absorption of iodine by the thyroid, so keep raw cabbage-family vegetables to a minimum to prevent reducing your production of thyroxine and, therefore, your metabolism. Nutritional experts estimate that about 20% of a healthful diet should consist of cooked produce for full nutritional benefit; the remaining 80% should be raw and whole (meaning processed as little as possible).

The best method for cooking produce is steaming. In contrast, boiling vegetables leaches vitamins into the water, which is then typically discarded. Microwaving may not be as safe as was once thought because photon bombardment in the microwave range is known to cause molecular changes in food that may damage proteins and vitamins. The health effects are still unknown.

Breads, Meats, and Root Vegetables

Cooking methods such as baking, roasting, grilling, and deep frying change molecular characteristics that may damage health. Browning breads and meats, though tasty, causes sugars in the meats and starches in baked goods to bind to proteins. This creates AGEs (Advanced Glycation End-products) in a process called *glycation* that not only occurs within the food, but in your body. *Glycation* causes cellular damage, accelerating the aging process and contributing to disease states such as type-2 diabetes. Glycation, in fact, is a major player in type-2 diabetes. Eating glycated foods on an infrequent basis (less than twice monthly) may cause no long-term effects if raw produce and water intake are optimal. Poaching or stewing meats helps to avoid glycation in the foods, as well as in your body.

Eating sugar frequently causes glycation within bodily tissues, which manifests as facial wrinkles and an aged, sagging appearance to the skin. Sugar-eaters age more rapidly than those who abstain. It shows on their faces.

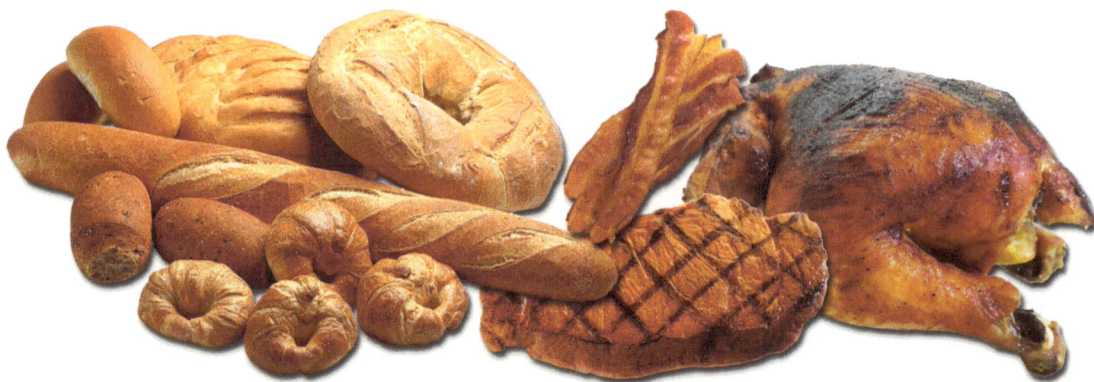

Grilling and Barbecuing

The outdoor barbecue has its own dangers. Not only AGEs, but PAHs (Polycyclic Aromatic Hydrocarbons) are created by grilling over a hot flame and smoking meats. PAHs are carcinogenic (cause cancer), mutagenic (damage DNA), and teratogenic (cause birth defects). Interestingly, marinating meats in beer, wine, or vinegar-based sauces ameliorates the effects of grilling by significantly reducing AGEs and PAHs. So, if you like to grill, don't forget to marinate!

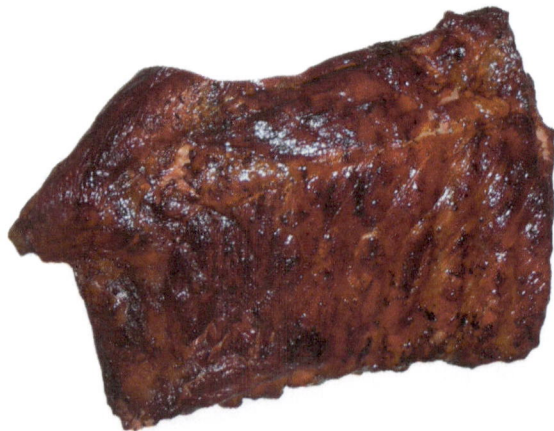

Eggs

Cooking eggs properly is an art, but also a science. The very nature of cooking an egg creates oxidation in the cholesterol portion of the egg—the yolk. *Cholesterol oxides* are the real culprits in evaluating the effects of dietary cholesterol on serum lipids. Scrambled, hard-boiled, and hard-frying eggs create the most cholesterol oxides. Cooking eggs so the yolk is still liquid is the most healthful, as in soft-boiled or sunny-side-up. Cooking meats and dairy products at high heat also creates cholesterol oxides, in addition to other chemicals damaging to health (the aforementioned AGEs and PAHs).

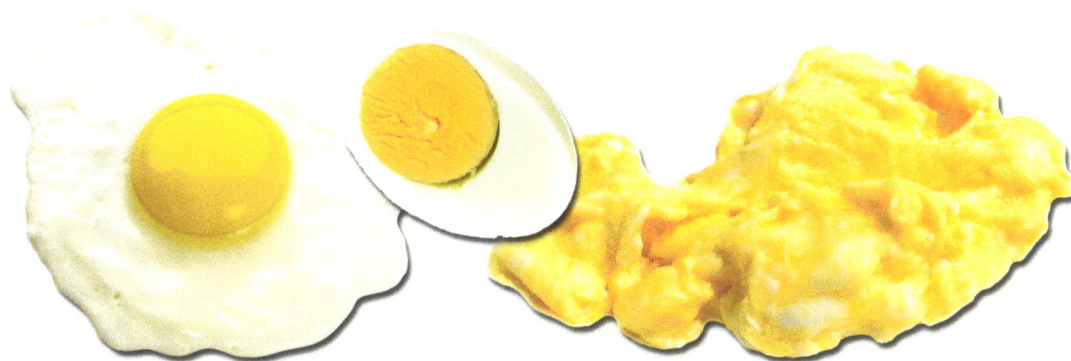

Fats in Baking

Recipes for baking typically require oils or butter, and these fats do not fare well at baking temperatures. As discussed earlier, at high temperatures, heated fats create free-radicals (unpaired electrons) that attack body cells, further creating PAHs (polycyclic aromatic compounds) that damage and age tissues.

The advent of almond flour looked like a boon for diabetics and others who needed a wheat-flour replacement, but we soon realized that high temperatures would create havoc with the fats inherent in the nut flour. The only safe baking flour is coconut flour.

Summary

A healthful diet means being kind to your food, eating 80% of your produce raw, and cooking meats and 20% of your produce slowly in stews and steam-pots. A weekly diversion into glycation hell will do minimal damage if you remember to marinate your meats and go easy on the grain products. It's okay to break the rules every once in a while. But most of the time, consuming as many raw foods as you can eat, and cooking with low, slow heat and lots of moisture are keys to keeping foods undamaged, so they don't damage *you*.

Nutrition Tables

For foods not listed, visit HTTP://WWW.CALORIEKING.COM
or HTTP://NUTRITIONDATA.SELF.COM/

Standard Serving Sizes

- Beverages, 1 cup
- Dairy, liquid, 1 cup
- Dairy, solidified, ½ cup
- Dry Cereals, ~1 cup (± ¼ cup)
- Grains, cooked, ½ cup
- Legumes, cooked, ½ cup

- Meats, 3½–4 ounces
- Nuts, 1 ounce (2 tablespoons)
- Vegetables, cooked, ½ cup
- Vegetables, raw, 1 cup
- Other, by piece

Composition of Selected Foods						
FOOD	QUANTITY	CALORIES	CARBS	PROTEIN	FAT	% FAT
DAIRY						
Butter	.5 oz (1 T)	99.00	0	0	11.00	100%
Cheese, American	1 oz	107.74	0.50	6.50	8.86	74%
Cheese, cheddar	1 oz	115.64	0.36	7.40	9.40	73%
Cheese, cottage, low-fat	4 oz	90.00	4.00	14.00	2.00	20%
Cheese, cottage, non-fat	4 oz	80.00	4.00	14.00	0.00	0%
Cheese, cottage, regular	4 oz	117.00	4.00	14.00	5.00	38%
Cheese, cream	1 oz	106.60	0.60	2.20	10.60	89%
Cheese, Monterey jack	1 oz	105.74	0.19	6.94	8.58	73%
Cheese, mozzarella, part-skim	1 oz	78.37	0.89	7.79	4.85	56%
Cheese, Parmesan, dry	1 oz	45.16	0.38	4.16	3.00	60%
Cheese, Swiss	1 oz	106.10	0.96	8.06	7.78	66%
Cream, half-and-half	1 oz	39.60	1.28	0.88	3.44	78%
Cream, heavy	1 oz	104.85	0.83	0.61	11.01	95%
Cream, substitute	1 oz	40.00	3.40	0.40	3.00	68%
Egg	1 large	79.20	0.30	6.00	6.00	68%
Egg Beaters	2 oz	30.00	1.00	6.00	0.00	0%
Ice cream	8 oz	274.70	31.70	4.80	14.3	47%
Ice milk	8 oz	187.31	29.00	5.16	5.63	27%
Milk, 2% fat	8 oz	121.40	11.70	8.12	4.68	35%
Milk, buttermilk	8 oz	124.20	11.70	8.10	5.00	36%
Milk, condensed sweet	8 oz	1002.60	166.00	24.80	26.60	24%

Composition of Selected Foods, continued						
FOOD	**QUANTITY**	**CALORIES**	**CARBS**	**PROTEIN**	**FAT**	**% FAT**
Milk, non-fat	8 oz	86.00	11.90	8.40	0.40	4%
Milk, whole 4% fat	8 oz	152.95	11.40	8.50	8.15	48%
Yogurt, plain low-fat	8 oz	143.28	16.00	11.90	3.52	22%
Yogurt, plain non-fat	8 oz	110.00	17.00	12.00	0.00	0%
Yogurt, plain whole-milk	8 oz	140.34	10.60	7.88	7.38	47%
MEATS						
Beef, dry chipped	3 oz	165.00	0	29.10	5.40	29%
Beef, ground supreme-lean (4% fat)	4 oz	177.17	0	34.19	4.49	23%
Beef, jerky	1 piece	38.00	1.40	4.20	1.70	40%
Beef, roast lean	4 oz	256.00	0	36.10	12.34	43%
Beef, short-ribs	4 oz	449.64	0	27.72	37.64	75%
Beef, steak porterhouse	4 oz	267.20	0	29.00	16.80	57%
Beef, steak round	4 oz	230.14	0	43.99	6.02	24%
Beef, steak sirloin	4 oz	228.40	0	28.93	12.52	49%
Beef, steak T-bone	4 oz	277.57	0	28.66	17.60	57%
Beef, tenderloin strip	4 oz	246.37	0	29.53	14.25	52%
Beef, veal cutlet	4 oz	306.02	0	37.94	17.14	50%
Franks, all meat	1 wiener	122.00	1.00	7.00	10.00	74%
Franks, turkey	1 wiener	100.00	0.60	5.80	8.10	73%
Lamb, chops	4 oz	245.66	0	30.86	13.58	50%
Lamb, leg roast	4 oz	210.16	0	31.21	9.48	41%
Lunch meat, bologna meat	1 slice	73.00	0.60	2.70	6.50	80%
Lunch meat, bologna turkey	1 slice	60.00	0.60	3.90	4.50	68%
Lunch meat, deviled ham	½ can	220.00	1.00	9.00	20.00	82%
Lunch meat, olive loaf	1 slice	67.00	2.60	3.40	4.70	63%
Lunch meat, pickle loaf	1 slice	74.00	1.70	3.30	6.00	73%
Lunch meat, salami beef	1 slice	57.40	0.60	3.40	4.60	72%
Lunch meat, turkey ham	1 slice	60.00	0.60	3.90	4.50	68%
Lunch meat, turkey pastrami	1 slice	40.00	0.50	5.20	1.80	38%
Pepperoni	1 slice	27.00	0.20	1.20	2.40	80%
Pork , ham cured	4 oz	256.51	0	28.56	15.63	55%
Pork, bacon	1 slice	34.70	0.10	1.60	3.10	80%
Pork, chops	4 oz	397.74	0	33.60	29.26	66%
Pork, roast	4 oz	218.17	0.00	20.14	15.29	63%
Pork, sausage	4 oz	412.65	1.23	22.32	35.37	77%
Pork, sirloin	4 oz	350.54	0.00	31.20	22.86	59%
Pork, spareribs	8 med	492.32	0	23.72	44.16	81%

Composition of Selected Foods, continued						
FOOD	QUANTITY	CALORIES	CARBS	PROTEIN	FAT	% FAT
Rabbit	4 oz	192.63	0	35.31	5.71	27%
Spam	1 oz	87.00	1.10	3.90	7.40	77%
Venison	4 oz	157.43	0	33.71	2.51	27%
POULTRY						
Chicken thigh fried	1 piece	162.00	2.00	16.60	9.30	52%
Chicken, breast fried	1 piece	153.70	1.00	28.80	4.10	24%
Chicken, breast no skin	1 piece	134.70	0	26.70	3.10	21%
Chicken, breast w/skin	1 piece	185.20	0	29.20	7.60	37%
Chicken, drum fried	1 piece	116.30	1.00	13.20	6.70	52%
Chicken, drum no skin	1 piece	72.50	0	12.50	2.50	31%
Chicken, drum w/skin	1 piece	108.60	0	14.10	5.80	48%
Chicken, gizzards	3.5 oz	146.50	1.10	27.20	3.70	23%
Chicken, ground breast	4 oz	140.00	0	32.00	3.50	23%
Chicken, livers	3.5 oz	150.70	0.90	24.40	5.50	33%
Chicken, thigh no skin	1 piece	109.00	0	13.50	5.70	47%
Chicken, thigh w/skin	1 piece	153.00	0	15.50	9.60	56%
Duck, no skin	4 oz	222.64	0	26.86	12.80	52%
Goose, no skin	4 oz	263.15	0	33.14	14.51	50%
Turkey, dark meat	4 oz	204.83	0	32.69	8.23	36%
Turkey, ground 10% fat	4 oz	185.31	0	34.00	5.00	24%
Turkey, white meat	4 oz	166.62	0	34.17	3.66	19%
SEAFOOD						
Bass	4 oz	107.14	0	21.43	2.38	20%
Caviar, sturgeon	1 tsp	26.00	3.30	2.70	1.50	52%
Clams, canned	4 oz	49.10	2.80	7.90	0.70	13%
Clams, fresh	9 small	78.30	8.30	14.00	1.90	22%
Cod	4 oz	87.27	0	19.95	0.83	9%
Crab, canned	4 oz	77.20	0.90	13.90	2.00	23%
Crab, fresh	4 oz	100.07	0.58	19.60	2.15	19%
Crab, fried	4 oz	185.00	8.60	10.70	12.00	58%
Fish cakes	4 oz	295.29	15.97	25.24	13.73	42%
Fish fillets, breaded	4 oz	311.00	20.00	11.00	23.00	67%
Fish sticks, fried	5	198.00	8.00	19.00	10.00	45%
Haddock	4 oz	89.75	0	20.75	0.75	8%
Halibut	4 oz	106.05	0	23.70	1.25	11%
Herring, pickled	3.5 oz	223.00	0	20.00	15.10	61%
Lobster	1 med tail	101.67	0.58	20.00	2.15	19%

Composition of Selected Foods, continued						
FOOD	**QUANTITY**	**CALORIES**	**CARBS**	**PROTEIN**	**FAT**	**% FAT**
Mackerel	4 oz	261.44	0	24.66	17.86	61%
Mussels, steamed	4 oz	108.57	3.77	16.46	2.51	21%
Oysters, canned	4 oz	76.15	4.10	10.10	2.15	25%
Oysters, fried	4 oz	273.14	11.43	23.20	12.34	41%
Perch	4 oz	111.02	0	21.50	2.80	23%
Red Snapper	4 oz	102.44	0	22.45	1.36	12%
Salmon, pink canned	4 oz	148.50	0	22.50	6.50	39%
Salmon, pink fresh	4 oz	238.80	0	25.50	15.20	57%
Salmon, sockeye canned	4 oz	159.55	0	23.35	7.35	41%
Sardines, canned in oil	1 oz	55.10	0	6.80	3.10	51%
Scallops, fresh	4 oz	87.47	4	17.35	0.23	2%
Scallops, fried	4 oz	210.26	11.43	20.57	9.14	39%
Shrimp, boiled	4 oz	97.02	1.70	20.53	0.90	9%
Shrimp, fried	4 oz	257.14	11.43	23.20	12.34	43%
Sole	4 oz	98.40	0	18.95	1.36	12%
Swordfish	4 oz	147.29	0	24.38	5.53	34%
Trout, rainbow	4 oz	238.86	0	23.54	15.31	58%
Tuna, albacore in oil	6.5 oz	381.00	0.10	50.60	19.90	47%
Tuna, albacore in water	6.5 oz	237.00	0	51.50	3.50	13%
Tuna, light in oil	6.5 oz	386.00	0.20	46.90	22.10	52%
Tuna, light in water	6.5 oz	202.50	0	45.00	2.50	11%
LEGUMES						
Beans, Garbanzo, cooked	1 cup	246.13	40.66	13.66	3.20	12%
Beans, Great Northern, cooked	1 cup	230.30	40.30	14.80	1.10	4%
Beans, kidney, cooked	1 cup	224.10	39.60	14.40	0.90	4%
Beans, lima, canned	1 cup	165.30	31.00	9.20	0.50	3%
Beans, pinto, cooked	1 cup	205.50	36.60	13.20	0.70	3%
Lentils, cooked	1 cup	216.80	38.60	15.60	0	0%
Peas, green, cooked	1 cup	117.40	19.40	8.60	0.60	5%
VEGETABLES						
Alfalfa sprouts	1 cup	45.80	5.00	5.10	0.60	12%
Artichoke	1 med	52.60	9.90	2.80	0.20	3%
Asparagus	4 spears	25.00	3.60	2.20	0.20	7%
Bamboo shoots	1 cup	45.08	6.90	3.47	0.40	8%
Beans, green, cooked	1 cup	37.90	6.80	2.00	0.30	7%
Beans, green raw	1 cup	41.40	7.80	2.10	0.20	4%
Beets, cooked	1 cup	68.60	15.00	1.70	0.20	3%

Composition of Selected Foods, continued						
FOOD	**QUANTITY**	**CALORIES**	**CARBS**	**PROTEIN**	**FAT**	**% FAT**
Broccoli, cooked	1 cup	51.70	0.70	4.80	0.50	9%
Brussels sprouts, cooked	1 cup	71.00	9.90	6.50	0.60	8%
Cabbage, raw	1 cup	19.70	3.80	0.9	0.10	5%
Carrots, raw	1 large	45.00	9.70	1.10	0.20	4%
Cauliflower, cooked	1 cup	34.70	5.10	2.90	0.30	8%
Celery, raw	2 stalks	12.90	2.00	1.00	0.10	7%
Corn, creamed, canned	1 cup	239.90	51.20	5.40	1.50	6%
Corn, fresh	1 ear	105.00	21.00	3.00	1.00	9%
Corn, kernel, canned	1 cup	159.70	32.70	4.30	1.30	7%
Cucumber	1 med	18.90	3.60	0.90	0.10	5%
Eggplant, cooked	1 cup	44.40	8.20	2.00	0.40	8%
Garlic	1 clove	4.58	0.90	0.20	0.02	4%
Lettuce, Boston	1 cup	9.30	1.40	0.70	0.10	10%
Lettuce, Iceberg	1 cup	12.50	2.20	0.70	0.10	7%
Lettuce, Romaine	1 cup	12.20	1.90	0.70	0.20	15%
Mushrooms, canned	8 oz	46.20	6.90	3.30	0.60	12%
Mushrooms, fresh	1 cup	21.80	3.10	1.90	0.20	8%
Okra, cooked	1 cup	55.70	9.60	3.20	0.50	8%
Olives, green	2 med	16.00	0.20	0.20	1.60	90%
Olives, ripe	2 med	19.60	0.30	0.10	2.00	92%
Onions, dry, raw	1 cup	71.40	14.80	2.60	0.20	3%
Onions, green	1 cup	40.60	8.20	1.50	0.20	4%
Parsley, fresh	1 cup	32.90	5.10	2.20	0.40	11%
Parsnips, cooked	1 cup	198.80	23.10	2.30	0.80	4%
Pepper, green bell	1 large	29.80	6.00	1.00	0.20	6%
Potato Buds, prepared	1 cup	268.00	34.00	6.00	12.00	40%
Potato chips	10	116.40	10.00	1.10	8.00	62%
Potato, baked	1 med	97.80	22.00	2.00	0.20	2%
Potatoes, French fries	10 large	139.80	18.00	2.10	6.60	42%
Potatoes, hash browns	8 oz	362.50	45.10	4.80	19.10	47%
Potatoes, mashed	1 cup	140.30	27.30	4.40	1.50	10%
Potatoes, mashed instant	1 cup	198.30	30.50	4.00	6.70	30%
Potatoes, scalloped w/cheese	1 cup	202.66	18.66	8.00	10.66	47%
Pumpkin, canned	1 cup	93.90	19.40	2.50	0.70	7%
Radishes	10 med	8.40	1.60	0.50	0	0%
Spinach, canned	1 cup	62.40	7.40	5.50	1.20	17%
Spinach, raw	1 cup	18.60	2.40	1.80	0.20	10%

Composition of Selected Foods, continued						
FOOD	QUANTITY	CALORIES	CARBS	PROTEIN	FAT	% FAT
Squash, summer	1 cup	30.60	5.60	1.60	0.20	6%
Squash, winter	1 cup	148.40	31.60	3.70	0.80	5%
Tomato paste	6 oz	150.00	35.00	6.00	0.50	3%
Tomato sauce	8 oz	80.00	13.00	3.00	0.50	6%
Tomato, raw	1 med	37.10	7.00	1.60	0.30	7%
Tomatoes, canned	1 cup	55.70	10.40	2.40	0.50	8%
Turnips, cooked	1 cup	37.90	7.60	1.20	0.30	7%
Yam, baked	1 cup	215.60	48.20	4.80	0.40	2%
Yeast, brewer's	1 T	25.70	3.10	3.10	0.10	4%
GRAIN PRODUCTS						
Biscuit	1—2"	102.80	12.80	2.10	4.80	42%
Bran, raw	1 cup	160.20	35.40	9.00	2.60	12%
Bread, corn	2" square	94.40	13.10	3.30	3.20	31%
Bread, French	1 slice	57.36	11.10	1.80	0.64	10%
Bread, pita	1	138.00	24.00	6.00	2.00	13%
Bread, raisin	1 slice	60.96	12.30	1.50	0.64	9%
Bread, rye	1 slice	59.10	12.00	2.10	0.30	5%
Bread, white enriched	1 slice	61.510	11.60	2.00	0.79	12%
Bread, whole wheat	1 slice	59.90	11.00	2.40	0.70	11%
Buns, hotdog or hamburger	1	117.80	21.20	3.30	2.20	17%
Corn meal	1 cup	430.40	88.00	10.60	4.00	8%
Cornflakes	1 cup	92.90	21.00	2.00	0.10	1%
Cracker, Cheezits	5	81.00	7.80	1.40	4.90	54%
Cracker, Melba toast	1	15.00	2.70	0.50	0.20	12%
Cracker, oyster	33	120.00	20.00	2.70	3.30	2%
Cracker, Ritz	1	17.33	1.83	0.20	1.00	52%
cracker, saltine	1	12.37	2.00	0.26	0.37	27%
Cracker, Triscuit	1	21.00	3.10	0.40	0.67	29%
Cracker, Waverly wafer	1	18.00	2.50	0.25	0.80	40%
Cracker, Wheat Thins	1	9.00	1.25	0.10	0.35	35%
Cream of Wheat cereal	1 cup	134.40	28.20	4.50	0.40	3%
Muffin, bran	1 muffin	116.30	17.20	3.10	3.90	30%
Muffin, English	1 muffin	129.00	25.20	4.50	1.10	8%
Noodles, chow mien	1 cup	306.00	31.60	5.40	17.60	52%
Noodles, pasta cooked	1 cup	197.20	37.30	6.60	2.40	11%
Noodles, Top Ramen cooked	1 cup	207.00	30.70	5.90	8.60	37%
Oatmeal, cooked	1 cup	134.00	23.30	4.80	2.40	16%

Composition of Selected Foods, continued						
Food	**Quantity**	**Calories**	**Carbs**	**Protein**	**Fat**	**% Fat**
Pancake, buckwheat	1—4" diam	55.30	6.40	1.80	2.50	41%
Pancake, white enriched	1—4" diam	53.50	7.20	1.90	1.90	32%
Popcorn, plain	1 cup	56.30	10.70	1.80	0.70	11%
Rice, brown cooked	1 cup	178.80	38.20	3.80	1.20	6%
Rice, white cooked	1 cup	218.40	49.60	4.10	0.40	2%
Roll, croissant	1	109.00	11.20	2.30	6.10	50%
Roll, dinner hard	1 med	112.60	20.10	3.10	2.20	18%
Shredded wheat	1 biscuit	94.50	20.00	2.50	0.50	5%
Tortilla, corn	1	65.40	13.50	1.50	0.60	9%
Tortilla, flour	1—9" diam	163.00	28.00	6.00	3.00	17%
Tortilla, taco shell	1	50.00	7.20	1.00	2.20	40%
Waffle	1—6" diam	207.00	28.10	7.00	7.40	32%
Wheat flakes	1 cup	129.00	24.20	3.10	2.20	15%
Fruits						
Apple	1 med.	99.00	240	0.30	0.20	2%
Applesauce	1 cup	112.10	26.40	0.50	0.50	4%
Apricot	1	19.72	4.56	0.37	0	0%
Avocado	1 med	362.40	12.60	4.20	32.80	81%
Banana	1 med	142.30	33.30	1.60	0.30	2%
Blackberries	1 cup	92.980	18.60	1.70	1.30	13%
Blueberries	1 cup	92.980	18.60	1.70	1.30	13%
Cantaloupe	½ med	65.60	15.00	1.40	0	0%
Cherries	1 cup	91.20	20.40	1.50	0.40	4%
Cranberry sauce, canned	1 cup	422.60	104.00	0.30	0.60	1%
Dates	10 med	304.90	72.90	2.20	0.50	1%
Figs	1	44.35	10.15	0.60	0.15	3%
Fruit cocktail	1 cup	207.50	50.20	1.00	0.30	1%
Grapefruit	1	92.20	21.60	1.00	0.20	2%
Grapes	1 cup	116.60	27.70	1.00	0.20	2%
Juice, apple	8 oz	118.8	29.50	0.20	0	0%
Juice, grapefruit	8 oz	98.60	23.00	1.20	0.20	2%
Juice, orange	8 oz	123.00	28.90	1.70	0.20	1%
Juice, tomato	8 oz	52.20	10.40	2.20	0.20	3%
Kumquat	1 med	12.00	3.20	0.20	0	0%
Lemon	1 med	29.00	6.00	0.80	0.20	6%
Lemonade, from concentrate	8 oz	113.60	28.30	0.10	0	0%
Mango	1 med	169.70	38.80	1.60	0.90	5%

Composition of Selected Foods, continued						
FOOD	**QUANTITY**	**CALORIES**	**CARBS**	**PROTEIN**	**FAT**	**% FAT**
Melon, cantaloupe	1	67.40	15.00	1.40	0.20	3%
Melon, honeydew	2" slice	55.30	11.50	1.20	0.50	8%
Melon, watermelon	1 cup	29.40	6.40	0.50	0.20	6%
Nectarine	1 med	97.60	23.60	0.80	0	0%
Orange	1 med	71.90	16.00	1.30	0.30	4%
Papaya	½ med	73.50	15.00	0.90	1.10	13%
Peach	1 med	42.10	9.70	0.60	0.10	2%
Pear	1	135.20	30.60	1.40	0.80	5%
Persimmon	1 medium	140.80	33.50	0.80	0.40	3%
Pineapple, raw	1 cup	89.90	21.20	0.60	0.30	3%
Plum	1 med	36.60	8.90	0.25	0	0%
Pomegranate	1 large	108.90	25.30	0.80	0.50	4%
Prunes	1 cup	454.60	108.00	3.40	1.00	2%
Raisins	1 cup	531.10	128.00	4.10	0.30	1%
Raspberries, red	1 cup	78.20	16.70	1.50	0.60	7%
Strawberries	1 cup	44.60	10.00	0.70	0.20	4%
Tangelo	1 med	39.70	9.20	0.50	0.10	2%
Tangerine	1 med	44.60	10.00	0.70	0.20	4%
NUTS AND SEEDS						
Almonds, raw	2 oz	227.37	6.93	6.60	19.25	76%
Almonds, roasted	2 oz	263.65	7.65	7.30	22.65	77%
Brazil nuts, raw	2 oz	271.10	38.25	5.00	10.90	36%
Cashews, roasted	2 oz	209.12	10.25	6.03	16.00	69%
Coconut meat, raw	1 cup	295.00	7.50	2.80	28.20	86%
Coconut meat, sweet	1 cup	358.76	33.00	2.24	24.20	61%
Macadamia nuts	6	116.90	1.50	1.40	11.70	90%
Peanut butter	1 T	101.30	3.20	3.90	8.10	72%
Peanuts, roasted	2 oz	225.21	7.43	9.43	17.53	76%
Pecans, raw	2 oz	198.79	3.95	2.48	19.23	87%
Pistachios	30 pieces	88.00	2.80	2.90	8.00	82%
Pumpkin seeds	2 oz	208.75	5.25	10.15	16.35	70%
Sesame seeds	2 oz	233.72	6.60	6.83	20.00	77%
Sunflower seeds	2 oz	218.07	7.23	8.70	17.15	71%
Walnuts, English raw	2 oz	174.60	3.95	3.70	16.00	82%
PROCESSED FOODS						
Banquet beef pie	8 oz	409.00	40.90	16.30	20.00	44%
Banquet chicken pie	8 oz	409.00	40.90	16.30	20.00	44%

Composition of Selected Foods, continued					
Food	Quantity	Calories	Carbs	Protein	Fat	% Fat
Banquet enchilada, beef	12 oz	479.00	63.60	17.00	17.30	33%
Banquet enchilada, cheese	12 oz	459.00	58.80	18.40	16.70	33%
Banquet fish dinner	8.75 oz	382.00	43.60	19.30	14.60	34%
Banquet macaroni and cheese	12 oz	386.00	45.60	13.30	10.20	24%
Banquet meatloaf dinner	10.75 oz	530.00	48.00	19.00	29.00	49%
Banquet meatloaf, Man Pleaser	19 oz	916.00	63.60	35.60	57.70	57%
Banquet Mexican combination	12 oz	521.00	41.00	22.00	30.00	52%
Banquet Salisbury steak	11 oz	390.00	24.00	18.10	24.60	57%
Banquet Salisbury steak, Man Pleaser	19 oz	873.00	71.70	37.70	48.00	49%
Banquet turkey dinner	11 oz	293.00	27.80	23.40	9.70	30%
Banquet turkey, Man Pleaser	19 oz	620.00	73.80	39.30	18.90	27%
Banquet veal parmagian	11 oz	421.00	42.10	20.60	19.00	41%
Bean dip, most brands	1 oz	33.00	2.90	1.50	1.10	30%
Campbell's Beans and Franks	8 oz	355.00	42.00	15.00	14.00	35%
Celeste pizza, cheese	¼ pizza	320.00	36.20	14.43	12.80	36%
Celeste pizza, deluxe	¼ pizza	367.00	33.90	16.20	18.60	46%
Celeste pizza, pepperoni	¼ pizza	356.00	31.70	16.30	18.20	46%
Celeste pizza, sausage	¼ pizza	375.00	33.90	16.00	19.50	47%
Cheetos	1 oz	159.00	15.40	1.80	10.00	57%
Chef Boyardee Beefaroni	7.5 oz	207.00	28.00	8.00	7.00	30%
Chef Boyardee Ravioli, beef	7.5 oz	210.00	32.00	7.00	6.00	26%
Chili con Carne w/beans	1 cup	327.00	30.00	18.00	15.00	41%
Chili con Carne, no beans	1 cup	506.00	15.00	26.00	38.00	68%
Cornflake crumbs, Kelloggs	1 oz	108.00	25.00	2.00	0	0%
CornNuts snack corn	1 oz	120.00	19.00	2.00	4.00	30%
Cracker jacks	1 oz	114.00	25.50	0.80	1.00	8%
Dinner Classics beef short ribs	10.5 oz	418.00	29.00	26.00	22.00	47%
Dinner Classics chicken/noodles	12 oz	354.00	30.00	27.00	14.00	36%
Dinner Classics Salisbury steak	11.5 oz	457.00	37.00	21.00	25.00	49%
Dinner Classics sirloin roast	11 oz	294.00	22.00	29.00	10.00	31%
Dinner Classics turkey/dressing	11.25 oz	33.000	32.0	19.0	14.00	38%
Doritos tortilla chips	1 oz	139.00	18.60	2.0	6.60	43%
Egg rolls, La Choy	4	117.00	14.40	3.8	4.20	32%
Fritos corn chips	1 oz	155.00	15.80	1.9	9.70	56%
Gravy, beef canned	½ can	77.00	7.00	5.4	3.40	40%
Gravy, brown from mix	4 oz	40.00	8.00	1.0	1.00	23%

Composition of Selected Foods, continued						
FOOD	QUANTITY	CALORIES	CARBS	PROTEIN	FAT	% FAT
Gravy, chicken canned	½ can	118.00	8.10	2.8	8.50	65%
Gravy, chicken from mix	4 oz	41.00	7.10	1.3	0.90	20%
Hamburger Helper beef noodle	⅕ pkg.	320.00	25.00	20.0	15.00	42%
Hamburger Helper beef Romanoff	⅕ pkg.	340.00	28.00	21.0	16.00	42%
Hamburger Helper cheeseburger mac	⅕ pkg.	360.00	28.00	21.00	16.00	51%
Hamburger Helper chili tomato	⅕ pkg.	320.00	29.00	19.00	14.00	39%
Hamburger Helper hash	⅕ pkg.	300.00	24.00	18.00	15.00	45%
Hamburger Helper lasagna	⅕ pkg.	330.00	33.00	19.00	14.00	38%
Hamburger Helper pizza bake	⅕ pkg.	340.00	33.00	20.00	14.00	37%
Hamburger Helper potato Stroganoff	⅕ pkg.	320.00	27.00	18.00	15.00	42%
Hamburger Helper potatoes au gratin	⅕ pkg.	320.00	27.00	18.00	15.00	42%
Hamburger Helper rice oriental	⅕ pkg.	340.00	35.00	18.00	14.00	37%
Hamburger Helper spaghetti	⅕ pkg.	330.00	31.00	20.00	14.00	38%
Hamburger Helper stew	⅕ pkg.	290.00	23.00	18.00	14.00	43%
Hamburger Helper tamale pie	⅕ pkg.	190.00	39.00	4.00	2.00	9%
Hash, corned beef	6 oz	288.00	12.00	24.00	16.00	50%
Le Menu sliced turkey	11.25 oz	464.00	34.00	28.00	24.00	47%
Macaroni and cheese, Kraft	6 oz	297.00	36.00	9.00	13.00	39%
Noodle Roni Parmesano, dry	1.2 oz	131.00	21.00	5.00	3.00	21%
Pork and beans	6 oz	246.00	37.00	11.00	6.00	22%
Pretzels	1 oz	111.00	22.40	2.6.00	1.00	8%
Soup, bean canned	1 cup	197.00	30.00	8.00	5.00	23%
Soup, chicken canned	1 cup	82.00	12.00	4.00	2.00	22%
Soup, cream of...canned	1 cup	208.00	18.00	7.00	12.00	52%
Soup, noodle; barley; rice	1 cup	112.00	13.00	6.00	4.00	32%
Soup, split pea canned	1 cup	159.00	25.00	8.00	3.00	17%
Soup, vegetable beef canned	1 cup	104.00	11.00	6.00	4.00	35%
Spaghetti and meat sauce canned	1 cup	282.00	35.00	13.00	10.00	32%
Stew, beef canned	1 cup	210.00	15.00	15.00	10.00	43%
Stouffer's French bread pizza, cheese	5.13 oz	330.00	43.00	10.00	13.00	35%
Stouffer's French bread pizza, deluxe	5.13 oz	400.00	46.00	15.00	18.00	41%
Stouffer's French bread pizza, pepperoni	5.13 oz	410.00	44.00	12.00	20.00	44%

Composition of Selected Foods, continued						
FOOD	QUANTITY	CALORIES	CARBS	PROTEIN	FAT	% FAT
Stouffer's lasagna	1	385.00	36.00	28.00	14.00	33%
Stovetop bread stuffing	1 cup	354.00	42.00	6.00	18.00	46%
Swanson beef dinner	15 oz	490.00	57.00	29.00	17.00	31%
Swanson beef lasagna	12.25 oz	490.00	54.00	25.00	20.00	37%
Swanson beef, Hungry Man	17 oz	540.00	51.00	44.00	18.00	30%
Swanson fried chicken dinner	15 oz	630.00	65.00	24.00	31.00	44%
Swanson ham dinner	10 oz	380.00	47.00	19.00	13.00	31%
Swanson Salisbury steak, Hungry Man	16 oz	490.00	47.00	23.00	23.00	42%
Swanson turkey dinner	16 oz	520.00	62.00	27.00	19.00	33%
Swanson turkey, Hungry Man	18.75 oz	740.00	79.00	48.00	26.00	32%
Swanson veal parmagiana	11 oz	421.00	42.10	20.60	19.00	41%
Tamales, canned	1	109.00	11.00	3.50	5.50	46%
Tuna Helper	⅕ pkg.	230.00	28.00	14.00	7.00	27%
Van de Kamps enchiladas, beef	4	342.00	33.00	16.00	16.00	42%
Van de Kamps enchiladas, chicken	7.5 oz	247.00	24.00	14.00	11.00	40%
Van de Kamps enchiladas, shred. beef	6 oz	214.00	20.00	12.00	10.00	42%
Van de Kamps fillet o' fish	12 oz	300.00	27.00	25.00	11.00	33%
Van de Kamps fish and chips	5 oz	290.00	25.00	13.00	15.00	47%
Van de Kamps microwave sole	5 oz	294.00	17.00	16.00	18.00	55%
CONDIMENTS						
Barbecue sauce	1 T	15.68	1.25	0.24	1.08	62%
Catsup	1 T	17.20	3.80	0.30	0.08	4%
Dressing, bleu cheese	1 T	77.40	1.10	0.70	7.80	91%
Dressing, bleu cheese lite	1 T	40.30	1.50	0.70	3.50	78%
Dressing, Italian	1 T	85.00	1.00	0	9.00	95%
Mayonnaise	1 T	102.80	0.30	0.20	11.20	98%
Oil, vegetable	1 T	126.00	0	0	14.00	100%
Sandwich spread	1 T	53.00	2.00	0	5.00	85%
Steak sauce	1 T	20.00	2.50	0	0	0%
Tartar sauce	1T	31.90	0.90	0.10	3.10	97%
BEVERAGES						
Awake citrus drink	6 oz	91.00	21.90	0.10	0.30	3%
Beer, Miller Lite	12 oz	96.00	2.80	0.90	0.80	8%
Beer, regular	12 oz	151.50	13.65	0.90	0.80	5%
Cola	12 oz	141.00	35.25	0	0	0

Composition of Selected Foods, continued						
FOOD	**QUANTITY**	**CALORIES**	**CARBS**	**PROTEIN**	**FAT**	**% FAT**
Gatorade	8 oz	39.00	10.50	0	0	0
Hawaiian Punch	8 oz	120.00	29.30	0.10	0	0
Kool-aid, w/sugar	8 oz	95.00	24.20	0	0	0
Tang	6 oz	87.00	22.20	0	0	0
Vodka, Gin, Rum 80 proof	1.5 oz	97.00	0	0	0	0
Whiskey, brandy 90 proof	1.5 oz	119.00	0	0	0	0
Wine, dry	4 oz	100.00	1.50	0	0	0
Wine, sweet	4 oz	165.00	9.20	0.12	0	0

Nutrition Values of Selected Fast Foods

KEY: Cals = Calories **C** = Carbohydrates **P** = Protein **F** = Fat **Na⁺** = Sodium

RESTAURANT	**FOOD ITEM**	**CALS**	**C**	**P**	**F**	**% F**	**NA⁺ MGS**
Arby's	Club sandwich	560	43	30	30	48%	1610
Arby's	Ham and cheese sandwich	380	23	33	17	40%	1350
Arby's	Roast beef sandwich	350	32	22	15	39%	980
Arby's	Super roast beef sandwich	620	61	30	28	41%	1420
Arby's	Turkey sandwich	510	46	28	24	42%	1220
Burger King	Apple pie	240	32	2	12	45%	335
Burger King	Chicken Tenders, 6	204	10	20	10	44%	636
Burger King	Chocolate shake	340	57	8	10	26%	280
Burger King	Double Beef Whopper	887	42	51	57	58%	922
Burger King	French fries, regular	227	24	3	13	52%	160
Burger King	Onion rings	270	29	3	16	53%	450
Burger King	Whopper with cheese	709	43	33	45	57%	1126
Carl's Jr.	California Roast Beef sandwich	300	34	25	7	21%	505
Carl's Jr.	Famous Star burger	530	38	24	32	54%	705
Carl's Jr.	Filet of Fish sandwich	570	61	20	27	43%	790
Carl's Jr.	French fries, regular	250	25	3	15	54%	460
Carl's Jr.	Onion rings	330	39	5	17	46%	75
Carl's Jr.	Super Star burger	780	38	43	50	58%	785
Dairy Queen	Buster Bar	240	37	10	22	83%	n/a
Dairy Queen	Cheese dog, super	593	43	26	36	55%	1986
Dairy Queen	Cheeseburger	318	30	18	14	40%	871
Dairy Queen	Chili dog	330	25	13	20	55%	937

Nutrition Values of Selected Fast Foods, continued							
RESTAURANT	FOOD ITEM	CALS	C	P	F	% F	NA⁺ MGS
Dairy Queen	Chili dog, super	555	42	23	33	54%	1640
Dairy Queen	Dilly Bar	240	22	4	15	56%	n/a
Dairy Queen	Hamburger	260	28	13	9	31%	572
Dairy Queen	Hamburger, big	457	37	27	23	45%	909
Dairy Queen	Hamburger, super	783	35	53	48	55%	1624
Dairy Queen	Hot dog	273	23	11	15	49%	868
Dairy Queen	Shake, large	840	125	22	28	30%	n/a
Domino's Pizza	12" pepperoni, 2 slices	380	48	20	12	28%	880
Domino's Pizza	12" cheese, 2 slices	340	52	18	6	16%	660
Domino's Pizza	16" cheese, 2 slices	400	58	24	8	18%	800
Domino's Pizza	16" pepperoni, 2 slices	440	56	24	14	29%	1080
Jack In The Box	Apple turnover	411	45	4	24	53%	352
Jack In The Box	Cheeseburger	310	28	16	15	44%	877
Jack In The Box	Chicken Supreme sandwich	601	39	31	36	54%	1582
Jack In The Box	Chocolate shake	325	55	11	7	19%	270
Jack In The Box	Fish Supreme sandwich	455	38	17	26	51%	837
Jack In The Box	French fries, regular	221	27	2	12	49%	164
Jack In The Box	Hamburger	263	29	13	11	38%	566
Jack In The Box	Jumbo Jack	551	45	28	29	47%	1134
Jack In The Box	Jumbo Jack with cheese	630	45	32	35	50%	1665
Jack In The Box	Onion rings	382	39	5	23	54%	403
Jack In The Box	Super Taco	288	21	12	17	53%	765
Jack In The Box	Taco, regular	191	16	8	11	52%	406
KFC	Coleslaw	121	13	9	8	60%	225
KFC	Extra-crispy breast	354	17	18	24	61%	79
KFC	Extra-crispy drumstick	173	6	13	11	57%	346
KFC	Kentucky Fries	268	33	5	13	43%	8
KFC	Kentucky Nuggets, 6	276	13	17	17	57%	840
KFC	Original Recipe breast	276	10	20	17	55%	654
KFC	Original Recipe drumstick	147	3	14	9	54%	261
KFC	Potatoes and gravy	87	14	2	3	31%	325
Long John Silver's	Batter-fried fish dinner	711	60	17	45	57%	1297
Long John Silver's	Batter-fried fish, 1 piece	202	11	13	12	53%	673
Long John Silver's	Chicken Nugget (6) dinner	699	54	23	45	58%	853
Long John Silver's	Chicken Plank	152	10	9	8	47%	515
Long John Silver's	Fried fish (3) dinner	1181	93	47	70	53%	2797
Long John Silver's	Fryes	247	31	4	12	44%	6

Nutrition Values of Selected Fast Foods, continued							
RESTAURANT	FOOD ITEM	CALS	C	P	F	% F	NA⁺ MGS
Long John Silver's	Hushpuppies, 2	145	18	3	7	43%	405
McDonald's	Big Mac	570	39	25	35	55%	979
McDonald's	Chicken McNuggets, 6	323	15	19	20	56%	512
McDonald's	Chocolate shake	383	66	10	9	21%	300
McDonald's	Egg McMuffin	327	31	19	15	41%	885
McDonald's	Filet o' Fish sandwich	432	37	14	25	52%	781
McDonald's	French fries, regular	220	26	3	12	49%	109
McDonald's	Hamburger	263	29	13	11	38%	566
McDonald's	McDLT	680	40	30	44	58%	1030
McDonald's	Quarter-pounder with cheese	525	31	30	32	55%	1220
Pizza Hut	½—10" beef, thick	620	73	38	20	29%	800
Pizza Hut	½—10" beef, thin	490	51	29	19	35%	800
Pizza Hut	½—10" cheese, thick	560	71	34	14	23%	600
Pizza Hut	½—10" cheese, thin	450	54	25	15	30%	600
Pizza Hut	½—10" pepperoni, thick	560	68	31	18	29%	800
Pizza Hut	½—10" pepperoni, thin	430	45	23	17	36%	800
Pizza Hut	½—10" sausage, thin	520	51	27	23	40%	800
Pizza Hut	½—10" supreme, thick	640	74	36	22	31%	800
Pizza Hut	½—10" supreme, thin	510	51	27	21	37%	800
Pizza Hut	½—10"sausage, thick	640	71	36	23	32%	800
Taco Bell	Bean burrito	350	48	15	11	28%	300
Taco Bell	Beef burrito	466	37	30	21	41%	327
Taco Bell	Beefy tostada	291	21	19	15	46%	138
Taco Bell	Burrito Supreme	457	43	21	22	43%	367
Taco Bell	Combination burrito	404	43	21	16	36%	300
Taco Bell	Enchirito	373	36	19	17	41%	1304
Taco Bell	Pintos n' Cheese	232	30	13	6	23%	101
Taco Bell	Taco, regular	162	9	12	9	50%	200
Taco Bell	Tostada	179	25	9	6	30%	101
Wendy's	Chicken sandwich	320	31	25	10	28%	500
Wendy's	Chili con carne	230	21	19	9	31%	1065
Wendy's	Chocolate shake	390	54	9	16	37%	247
Wendy's	Double hamburger	560	24	41	34	55%	575
Wendy's	french fries, regular	280	35	4	14	45%	95
Wendy's	Taco salad	390	36	23	18	42%	1100
Wendy's	Triple cheeseburger	1040	35	72	68	59%	1848

Nutrition Value of Selected Dry Breakfast Cereals (1 oz)						
COMPANY	PRODUCT	CALORIES	FIBER	PROTEIN	ADDED SUGAR	SODIUM
Kellogg's	All Bran	70	9	4	5	270
Kellogg's	Apple Jacks	110	t	2	14	125
Ralston/Purina	Bran Chex	90	5	3	5	300
General Mills	Cheerios	110	2	4	1	330
Post	Cocoa Pebbles	110	t	1	12	150
General Mills	Cocoa Puffs	110	t	1	4	200
Quaker	Corn Bran	110	5	2	6	300
Ralston/Purina	Corn Chex	110	t	1	12	310
Kellogg's	Corn Flakes	110	t	2	2	280
Kellogg's	Corn Pops	110	t	1	12	90
Kellogg's	Cracklin' Oat Bran	120	4	3	8	190
Kellogg's	Crispix	110	t	2	3	220
General Mills	Crispy Wheats & Raisins	110	t	2	10	180
General Mills	Fiber One	60	12	3	2	220
Kellogg's	Frosted Flakes	110	t	1	11	190
Kellogg's	Frosted Mini Wheats	110	3	3	6	5
Post	Fruit & Fiber, tropical	90	4	2	6	160
Kellogg's	Fruit Loops	110	t	2	13	125
General Mills	Golden Grahams	120	t	1	12	220
Post	Grape Nuts	110	2	3	3	190
Post	Grape Nuts Flakes	100	2	3	5	170
Post	Honey Comb	110	t	1	11	180
General Mills	Honey Nut Cheerios	110	t	3	10	255
Kellogg's	Honey Smacks	110	t	2	16	70
Kellogg's	Kocoa Krispies	110	t	1	10	190
Quaker	Life	120	1	5	6	180
General Mills	Lucky Charms	110	t	2	11	180
Post	Natural Bran Flakes	90	5	3	5	230
Post	Natural Raisin Bran	90	4	2	9	160
Kellogg's	Nutri Grain Wheat	110	2	3	2	195
Kellogg's	Nutri Grain Corn	110	2	2	2	185
Kellogg's	Product 19	110	t	2	3	290
Kellogg's	Raisin Bran	80	4	2	9	150
Ralston/Purina	Rice Chex	110	t	1	2	280
Kellogg's	Rice Crispies	110	t	2	3	280
Nabisco	Shredded Wheat	110	3	3	0	t

Nutrition Value of Selected Dry Breakfast Cereals (1 oz), continued						
COMPANY	PRODUCT	CALORIES	FIBER	PROTEIN	ADDED SUGAR	SODIUM
Nabisco	Shredded Wheat and Bran	110	4	3	0	0
Kellogg's	Special K	110	t	6	3	230
Post	Super Golden Crisp	110	t	2	14	45
General Mills	Total	130	2	3	3	280
Ralston/Purina	wheat Chex	100	2	3	2	200
General Mills	Wheaties	110	2	3	3	370

Nutrition Value of Selected Desserts (Sweets, Confections)							
FOOD	AMOUNT	CALS	C	P	F	% C	% F
Almond Joy	1 oz	151.00	18.5	1.70	7.80	49%	46%
Animal Crackers	15	120.00	22.0	1.90	2.90	73%	22%
Brownies	1 average	153.80	15.3	2.00	9.40	40%	55%
Brownies, Turtle, Duncan Hines	1/15 package	238.00	34.0	3.00	10.00	57%	38%
Cake, angel food	1/10 cake	122.10	27.1	3.20	0.10	89%	1%
Cake, devil's food, plain	1/10 cake	171.70	23.40	2.20	7.70	55%	40%
Chocolate Kisses	6	154.00	15.90	2.10	9.00	41%	53%
Chocolate peanuts	1 oz	153.00	13.30	4.60	9.00	35%	53%
Chocolate raisins	1 oz	115.00	19.50	1.00	3.70	68%	29%
Chocolate syrup	1 T	53.10	11.70	0.45	0.50	88%	8%
Cookie, chocolate chip	1	51.00	6.00	0.55	3.00	47%	53%
Cookie, oatmeal	1	80.00	12.20	1.10	3.20	61%	36%
Cookie, Oreo	1	49.00	7.10	0.50	2.10	58%	39%
Cookie, vanilla wafer	1	17.120	2.73	0.20	0.60	64%	32%
Doughnut, raised	1	124.80	11.30	1.89	8.00	36%	58%
Fig Bar	1	51.40	10.50	0.55	0.80	82%	14%
Graham cracker, chocolate covered	1	62.00	8.80	0.70	3.10	57%	43
Hard candy	6 pieces	108.00	27.20	0	0.30	100%	0%
Hershey's milk chocolate	1.02 oz	160.00	16.50	2.20	9.40	41%	53%
Hershey's Special Dark	1.02 oz	157.00	17.90	1.70	7.80	46%	45%
Hostess cupcakes, chocolate	2	314.00	58.80	2.90	8.80	75%	25%
Hostess Snoballs	2	269.00	49.60	2.50	7.60	74%	25%
Jam, preserves	1 T	56.40	14.00	0.10	0	99%	1%
Jello, sugar free	1 cup	8.00	0	2.00	0	0%	0%
Kit Kat	1.5 oz	210.00	25.00	3.00	11.00	48%	47%
Life Savers	5 pieces	39.00	9.7.0	0.00	0.10	100%	0%

Nutrition Value of Selected Desserts (Sweets, Confections), continued							
FOOD	AMOUNT	CALS	C	P	F	% C	% F
M & Ms	1.59 oz	220.00	31.00	3.00	10.00	56%	41%
M & Ms, peanut	1.67 oz	240.00	28.00	5.00	12.00	47%	45%
Mars bar	1.7 oz	230.00	29.00	4.00	10.00	52%	39%
Mounds	1 oz	147.00	19.90	1.20	6.90	54%	42%
Mr. Goodbar	1.27 oz	198.00	17.60	4.70	11.90	36%	54%
Nestle's Crunch	1.06 oz	160.00	19.00	2.00	8.00	48%	45%
Pie, apple	⅛—9" pie	417.80	61.00	3.40	17.80	58%	38%
Pie, Boston cream	⅛—9" pie	313.70	51.40	5.20	9.70	66%	28%
Pie, pumpkin	⅛—9" pie	322.00	36.70	6.00	16.80	46%	47%
Popsicle	1	65.00	16.70	0	0	100%	0
Pudding, chocolate	1 cup	409.40	66.80	8.10	12.20	65%	27%
Pudding, Jello sugar free	1 cup	164.00	26.00	8.00	4.00	63%	22%
Reese's Peanut Butter Cup	1 oz	184.00	17.40	4.40	10.70	38%	52%
Rolo	5 pieces	139.00	19.00	1.30	6.40	55%	41%
Sherbet	1 cup	236.00	57.60	2.80	0	98%	0
Smuckers butterscotch topping	1 T	70.5	16.50	0	0.50	94%	6%
Snickers	2 oz	270.00	33.00	6.00	13.00	49%	43%
Three Musketeers	2.28 oz	280.00	49.00	2.00	80	70%	26%
Twix	1.73 oz	120.00	16.00	1.00	60	53%	45%

Supplements That Lower Blood Glucose

This list of supplements—vitamin, mineral, and herbal products—have been extensively tested and are useful in controlling/lowering and treating tissue damage from high blood glucose. Use of these compounds is recommended *only with the guidance of a qualified health professional* (doctor, nutritionist, or medical dietician) and frequent in-home blood glucose testing to assess the effects of the products. These products may be mixed, but individual dosage adjustments are critical. *Extreme care in blood sugar monitoring* must accompany the multi-supplement approach.

WARNING: These products can cause a precipitous drop in blood sugar that may be life-threatening if used without frequent blood-sugar testing. Use of these products in combination with medically prescribed medications is recommended *only* under a doctor's supervision. Taking these products while fasting may result in an emergency situation requiring medical intervention.

PRODUCT	THERAPEUTIC DOSE	HOW OFTEN	COMMENTS
VITAMINS & MINERALS			
Biotin	1000 mcg (1 extra-strength tablet)	2x daily	Take with food.
Chromium Polynicotinate	500 mcg (1 extra-strength capsule)	2x daily	Take with food. May substitute *picolinate* form, but is slightly less bioavailable than polynicotinate form.
Vanadyl Sulfate (vanadium)	50 mg (5 tablets)	2x daily	Vanadyl sulfate tablets are available in maximum doses of 10 mg, so up to ten tablets must be taken daily. This mineral may cause a harmless darkening of the stool, and abdominal cramps/diarrhea/nausea in some individuals.
Benfotiamine (fat-soluble thiamine— vitamin B1)	160 mg (1 capsule)	2x daily	Take with food. This vitamin will not lower blood sugar. Benfotiamine is extraordinary in preventing and treating nerve/eye/organ damage from high blood sugar by increasing production of the *transketolase* enzyme that prevents glucose from converting to damaging sorbitol—a sugar alcohol.

Supplements That Lower Blood Glucose, continued			
Product	**Therapeutic Dose**	**How Often**	**Comments**
Vitamins & Minerals			
Alpha Lipoic Acid (ALA)	600 mg (1 extra-strength capsule)	2x daily	Take with food. May cause heartburn with too little food. Prevents and reverses damage to nerves, blood vessels, and organs due to hyperglycemia.
Magnesium Citrate	100 mg (1 capsule)	3x daily	Take with food. This mineral is critical in metabolizing glucose. Take in proper ratio with Calcium (50% of calcium intake).
Herbs & Spices			
Cinnamon (*Cinnamomum cassia*)	2000 mg (4 capsules)	3x daily	Take with food, or on empty stomach to reduce fasting glucose levels. Cinnamon contains *type-A polymers* that activate *kinase receptors*, increasing insulin sensitivity in cells. Very effective at reducing high fasting glucose. Cinnamon contains *coumarin*—a blood thinner; use caution when taking with aspirin or anticoagulant medications.
Gymnema sylvestre	800 mg (2 caplets)	2x daily	Take 30 minutes before meals. An herb known to not only lower blood glucose, but dull the sensation of sweet tastes.
Fenugreek (*Trigonella foenum-graecum*)	1200 mg (2 capsules)	3x daily	Take 30 minutes before meals.
Glucomannan (Konjac root)	1400 mg (2 capsules)	3x daily	Take 30 minutes before meals with a full glass of water. Glucomannan is a fiber that stimulates intestinal cells to produce fat-metabolizing hormones.
Banaba Leaf (*Lagerstroemia speciosa*)	400 mg (1 capsule)	2x daily	Take 30 minutes before meals. Very effective at lowering blood glucose, so use caution and test your blood sugar.
Bitter Melon (*Momordica charantia*)	1000 (2 capsules)	2x daily	Take with food. Very effective at lowering blood glucose, so use caution and test your blood sugar.

Supplements That Lower Blood Glucose, continued			
PRODUCT	**THERAPEUTIC DOSE**	**HOW OFTEN**	**COMMENTS**
HERBS & SPICES			
Berberine (*Berberis aristata*)	800 mg (2 capsules)	2x daily	Take with food. Exceptional at lowering post-meal glucose surges. Use caution and test your blood sugar.
Ivy Gourd (*Coccinia cordifolia*)	400 mg (1 capsule)	3x daily	Take 30 minutes before meals. Use caution and test your blood sugar.
Purslane (Portusana®) (*Portulaca oleracea*)	60 mg (1 capsule)	3x daily	Take 30 minutes before meals.
Indian Kino Tree (Silbinol®) (*Pterocarpus marsupium*)	150 mg (1 capsule)	3x daily	Take 30 minutes before meals.
African Mango (*Irvingia gabonensis*)	600 mg 2 capsules	2x daily	Take with food. African mango is *thermogenic* and raises metabolism slightly. May be useful in weight loss.
Green Coffee Bean extract (*Caffea canephora*)	200 mg (1 capsule)	2x daily	Take with food. Green coffee beans are *thermogenic* and raise metabolism slightly. May be useful in weight loss.

Supplements That Raise Blood Glucose

- Therapeutic doses of **niacin** (2000 or more mgs daily), used to lower cholesterol, may increase blood glucose in some individuals.

- Omega-3 supplements in the form of **fish oil** may increase blood glucose in some individuals.

- *Arginine and ornithine*—amino acids useful in promoting the production of human growth hormones—have been shown to raise blood glucose. If you have hyperglycemic episodes or diabetes, do not use these amino acids.

Recommended YouTube Videos
on Nutrition and Endocrinology

Donald W. Miller, Jr., M.D. *Enjoy Eating Saturated Fats: They're Good for You.*

HTTP://WWW.YOUTUBE.COM/WATCH?V=VRE9Z32NZHY&LIST=WL260CCD90493833A4

Gary Taubes at OSUMC (Ohio State University Medical Center): *Why We Get Fat*

- HTTP://WWW.YOUTUBE.COM/WATCH?V=BTUSPJZG-WC

Gary Taubs, PhD: WWW.JUMPSTARTMD.COM
(Why We Get Fat; Good Calories, Bad Calories)

- HTTP://WWW.YOUTUBE.COM/WATCH?V=HEWC5FL04O0&LIST=WL260CCD90493833A4&INDEX=61
- HTTP://WWW.YOUTUBE.COM/WATCH?V=-MEOL6VYLHA&LIST=WL260CCD90493833A4&INDEX=62
- HTTP://WWW.YOUTUBE.COM/WATCH?V=OQPMJHEEW4S&LIST=WL260CCD90493833A4&INDEX=63

Robert Lustig, MD: WWW.JUMPSTARTMD.COM *(Sugar is a Toxin)*

- HTTP://WWW.YOUTUBE.COM/WATCH?V=9-BEDX5ACTM&LIST=WL260CCD90493833A4&INDEX=64
- HTTP://WWW.YOUTUBE.COM/WATCH?V=AQMWXIORUIY&LIST=WL260CCD90493833A4&INDEX=65
- HTTP://WWW.YOUTUBE.COM/WATCH?V=REPKKMDH1UA&LIST=WL260CCD90493833A4&INDEX=66
- HTTP://WWW.YOUTUBE.COM/WATCH?V=UCKHN1DJ-CE&LIST=WL260CCD90493833A4&INDEX=67
- *Sugar: The Bitter Truth:* HTTP://WWW.YOUTUBE.COM/WATCH?V=0Z5X0I92OZQ

Peter Attia, MD: WWW.JUMPSTARTMD.COM *(The Role of Fat in Weight Loss)*

- HTTP://WWW.YOUTUBE.COM/WATCH?V=VIEDYBGJSMQ&LIST=WL260CCD90493833A4
- HTTP://WWW.YOUTUBE.COM/WATCH?V=C3E0PFL370Y
- HTTP://WWW.YOUTUBE.COM/WATCH?V=JH5WQUZBTAY

William Davis, MD: *(Wheat Belly: The Unhealthy Whole Grain)*

- HTTP://YOUTU.BE/UBBURNQYVZW
- HTTP://YOUTU.BE/-JSI3RLWZ48

References

"Arachidonic acid and lipoxygenase products stimulate gonadotropin alpha-subunit mRNA levels in pituitary alpha T3-1 cell line: role in gonadotropin releasing hormone action," *Biochemistry*, 33: 12795–12799, United States, November 1, 1994

"Associations between insulin sensitivity, and free fatty acid and triglyceride metabolism independent of uncomplicated obesity," *Metabolism*, 43: 1275–1281, United States, October, 1994

"Diets rich in lean beef increase arachidonic acid and long-chain omega 3 polyunsaturated fatty acid levels in plasma phospholipids," *Lipids*, 29: 337–343, United States, May 1994

"Effect of dietary omega-3 and omega-6 polyunsaturated fatty acids on lipid-metabolizing enzymes in obese rat liver," *Lipids*, 29: 481–489, United States, July 1994

"Effects of low-dose fish oil concentrate on angina, exercise tolerance time, serum triglycerides, and platelet function, *Angiology*, 45: 1023–1031, United States, December, 1994

"Epidemiology of colorectal cancer revisited: are serum triglycerides and/or plasma glucose associated with risk?" *Cancer Epidemiol. Biomarkers Prev.*, 3: 687–695, United States, December, 1994

"Evidence that homocysteine is an independent risk factor for atherosclerosis in hyperlipidemic patients," *American Journal of Cardiology*, 75: 132–136, United States, January 15, 1995

"Fatty acid oxidation and cardiac function in the sodium pivalate model of secondary carnitine deficiency," *Metabolism*, 44: 499–505, United States, April 1995

"Hyperinsulinism in normotensive offspring of hypertensive patients, *Hypertension*, 23: I12–I15, United States, January, 1994

"In vivo and in vitro effects of gamma-linoleic acid and eicosapentaenoic acid on prostaglandin production and arachidonic acid uptake by human endometrium," *Prostaglandins, Leukotrienes, and Essential Fatty Acids*, 50: 321–329, Scotland, June 1994

"Influence of indomethacin and prostaglandins," *Prostaglandins, Leukotrienes, and Essential Fatty Acids*, 51: 41–45, Scotland, July 1994

"Insulin regulation of triacylglyerol-rich lipoprotein synthesis and secretion," *Biochimica et Biophysica. Acta*, 1215: 9–32, Netherlands, November 17, 1994

"Interactions of cytokines and lipid mediators in acute and chronic inflammation," *Int. Arch Allergy Immunol.*, 107: 3838–384, Switzerland, May–Jun, 1995

"L-propionyl carnitine protects erythrocytes and low density lipoproteins against peroxidation, *Drugs Exp. Clin. Res.,* 20: 191–197, Switzerland, 1994

"Molecular mechanism of acute ammonia toxicity and of its prevention by L-carnitine," *Adv. Exp. Med. Biol.,* 368: 65–77, United States, 1994

"Physiologic and pathologic roles of prostaglandins and other eicosanoids in bone metabolism," *Journal of Nutrition,* 125: 2024S–2027S, United States, July 1995

"Secondary causes of hyperlipemia," *Med. Clin. North. Am.,* 78: 117–141, United States, January 1994

"The effect of L-carnitine, administered through intravenous infusion of glucose, on both glucose and insulin levels in healthy subjects, *Drugs Exp. Clin. Res.,* 20: 257–262, Switzerland, 1994

ADA. *Position of the American Dietetic Assoc.: Vegetarian Diets.* Journal of the American Dietetic Assoc, 1993, 93:1317–1319

Ahima, R. S. et al. "Role of leptin in the neuroendocrine response to fasting," *Nature* 382, 250–252

Ahmad F, Khan MM, Rastogi AK, Chaubey M, Kidwai JR. "Effect of (-)epicatechin on cAMP content, insulin release and conversion of proinsulin to insulin in immature and mature rat islets in vitro," *Indian J Exp Biol.* 1991 Jun;29(6):516–20.

Anderson RA, Broadhurst CL, Polansky MM, Schmidt WF, Khan A, Flanagan VP, Schoene NW, Graves DJ. "Isolation and characterization of polyphenol type-A polymers from cinnamon with insulin-like biological activity," *J Agric Food Chem.* 2004 Jan 14;52(1):65–70.

Anderson, Jean, MS and Deskins, Barbara, PhD, RD. *The Nutrition Bible.* 1995

Atkins, Robert C. *Dr. Atkins' Diet Revolution,* Bantam Books, 1972

————. *Dr. Atkins' Nutrition Breakthrough,* Bantam Books, 1981

————. *Dr. Atkins' Superenergy Diet,* Bantam Books, 1977

Balch, James F. MD, and Balch, Phyllis A. CNC. *Prescription for Nutritional Healing A-Z Guide to Supplements.* Avery Publishing Group, Inc., 1998

Ballentine, Rudolph. *Diet and Nutrition: A Holistic Approach,* Himalayan International Institute, 1978

Barnard, Christiaan *The Body Machine,* Multi Media, 1981

Barroso, I. et al. "Dominant negative mutations in human PPARg associated with severe insulin resistance, diabetes mellitus, and hypertension," *Nature* 402, 880–883 (1999).

Bender, D. A. *Nutritional Biochemistry of the Vitamins.* 1992

Bianch, C. Paul, and Hilf, Russell. *Protein Metabolism and Biological Function.* 1970

Bianchini F, Kaaks R, Vainio H. "Overweight, obesity, and cancer risk," The Lancet: Oncology 2002;3(9): 565–74.

Biggs, Matthew. *Matthew Biggs's Complete Book of Vegetables.* 1997

Biology Today, Communications Research Machines, Inc., 1972

Boden, G. "Role of fatty acids in the pathogenesis of insulin resistance and NIDDM," *Diabetes* 46, 1–10 (1997).

Braverman, Eric, R., MD with Pfeiffer, Carl C., MD, PhD. *The Healing Nutrients Within.* 1987

Brewster, L. and Jacobson M. *The Changing American Diet: A Chronicle of American Eating Habits from 1910 to 1980,* Center for Science in the Public Interest, 1983

Brody, Jane. *Jane Brody's Nutrition Book,* W.W. Norton & Co., 1981

Brown, Henry, MD. *Protein Nutrition.* 1974

Burtis, C. Edward. *Nature's Miracle Medicine Chest.* 1971

Canadian International Grains Institute. *Grains and Oilseeds: Handling, Marketing, Processing.* 3RD Edition. Rev. 1982

Carper, Jean. and Krauss, Patricia, *Carbohydrate Gram Counter,* Bantam Books, 1973

————. *The Food Pharmacy,* Bantam Books, 1988

Chaitow, Leon ND, DO. *Thorsons Guide to Amino Acids.* 1991

Chapman and Mitchell. "The Physiology of Exercise," *Scientific American,* May 1965

Chawla, A., Schwarz, E. J., Dimaculangan, D. D. & Lazar, M. A. "Peroxisome proliferator-activated receptor g (PPARg): Adipose predominant expression and induction early in adipocyte differentiation," *Endocrinology* 135, 798–800 (1994).

Chen, Ke, et al, "Induction of leptin resistance through direct interaction of C-reactive protein with leptin," *Nature Medicine* 2006;12,425–432

Cheraskin, E., MD, DMD; Ringsdorf, William, Jr. DMD; and Clark, J.W., DDS. *Diet and Disease.* 1987

Chopra, J. G. et al: "Protein in the US Diet." *Journal of American Dietetic Association,* 72:253–58, 1978

Clark, Linda. *Secrets of Health and Beauty,* Jove Books, 1969

Claudio, Virginia S., and Lagua, Rosalinda T. *Nutrition and Diet Therapy Dictionary.* 3RD Edition. 1991

Cooper, Dr. Kenneth H. *Advanced Nutritional Therapies.* 1996

Crujeiras, A. et al. "Weight Regain after a Diet-Induced Loss Is Predicted by Higher Baseline Leptin and Lower Ghrelin Plasma Levels," *Journal of Clinical Endocrinology and Metabolism (JCEM)* 2010 95: 5037–5044

Cyborski, Cathy Kpica. "Protein Supplements and Body Building Programs." *Journal of American Medical Association,* 240 (1978):481

Davis, Adelle. *Let's Eat Right to Keep Fit,* Signet Books, 1954

————. *Let's Get Well,* Signet Books, 1965

Diamond, Harvey and Marilyn. *Fit For Life.* 1985

Donsbach, Kurt W. *Nutrition in Action,* Nutrition Consultants Association, 1980

————. *Nutritional Approach to Superhealth,* International Institute of Natural Health Sciences, 1980

Dulbecco, Renato, editor. *Encyclopedia of Human Biology.* 7 volumes. 1991

Dyck D., "Leptin Sensitivity in Skeletal Muscle is Modulated by Diet and Exercise," *Exerc. Sport Sci.* Rev. 2005; Vol. 33, No. 4, pp. 189–194.

Eagles, J.A. and Randall, M.N. *Handbook of Normal and Therapeutic Nutrition,* Raven Press, 1980

Eaton, S.B. "The ancestral human diet: what was it and should it be a paradigm for contemporary nutrition?" The Proceedings of the Nutrition Society 2006;65(1): 1–6.

Ensminger, Audrey; Ensminger, M.E.; Konlande, James E; and Robson, John R.K. *Concise Encyclopedia of Foods and Nutrition.* 1995

Erasmus, Udo. *Fats that Heal, Fats that Kill.* 1993

FAO/WHO/UNO (United Nations Organization). "Energy and protein requirements," *WHO Tech. Rep.* ser. no. 724, 1985

Fleck, Henrietta. *Introduction to Nutrition,* Macmillan Publishing Company, 1981

Friedman, J. M. & Halaas, J. L. "Leptin and the regulation of body weight in mammals," *Nature* 395, 763–770 (1998).

Garrison, Robert H. and Somer, Elizabeth. *Nutrition Desk Reference,* Keats Publishing Co., 1985

Goldbeck, Nikki and David. *American Wholefoods Cuisine.* 1983

Goodhart, R.S. and Shils, M.E. *Modern Nutrition in Health and Disease,* Lea and Febinger, 1980

Greer, Rita and Woodward, Dr. Robert. *The Book of Vitamins and Healthfood Supplements.* 1995

Griffith, H. Winter, MD. *Vitamins, Herbs, Minerals, and Supplements.* Rev. Ed. 1998

Gruberg, Edward and Raymond, Stephen. "Beyond Cholesterol," *Atlantic Monthly*, May, 1978

Hamilton, E.M.N. and Whitney, E.N. *Nutrition Concepts and Controversies,* West Publishing Co., 1982

Hannan JM, Ali L, Rokeya B, Khaleque J, Akhter M, Flatt PR, Abdel-Wahab YH. "Soluble dietary fibre fraction of *Trigonella foenum-graecum* (fenugreek) seed improves glucose homeostasis in animal models of type 1 and type 2 diabetes by delaying carbohydrate digestion and absorption, and enhancing insulin action," *Br J Nutr.* 2007 Mar;97(3):514–21.

Heinerman, John, PhD. *Dr. Heinerman's Encyclopedia of Nature's Vitamins and Minerals.* 1998

Hendler, Sheldon Saul, MD, PhD. *The Doctor's Vitamin and Mineral Encyclopedia.* 1990

Hermann R, Niebch G, Borbe HO, et al. "Enantioselective pharmacokinetics and bioavailability of different racemic alpha-lipoic acid formulations in healthy volunteers," *Eur J Pharm Sci.* 1996;4:167–174.

Hlebowicz J, Darwiche G, Bjorgell O and Almer LO. "Effect of cinnamon on postprandial blood glucose, gastric emptying, and satiety in healthy subjects," *Am J Clin Nutr* 2007; 85: 1552–1556.

Holford, Patrick. *Six Weeks to Superhealth.* 2000

Hotamisligil, G. S. "The role of TNFa and TNF receptors in obesity and insulin resistance," *J. Int. Med.* 245, 621–625 (1999).

Hunter, Beatrice Trum. *The Great Nutrition Robbery.* 1978.

Huyser, Earl S. *General College Chemistry,* D.C. Heath and Company, 1974

Jacob S, Rett K, Henriksen EJ, Haring HU. "Thioctic acid—effects on insulin sensitivity and glucose-metabolism," *Biofactors.* 1999;10(2-3):169–174.

Jacobson, Michael F. and Fritschner, Susan. *The Fast Food Guide,* Workman Publishing, 1986

Jarvill-Taylor KJ, Anderson RA, Graves DJ. "A-hydroxychalcone derived from cinnamon functions as a mimetic for insulin in 3T3-L1 adipocytes," *J Am Coll Nutr.* 2001 Aug;20(4):327–36.

Journal of Clinical Endocrinology and Metabolism (JCEM), 2004 89 2: 447–452 HTTP://JCEM. ENDOJOURNALS.ORG/CONTENT/89/2/447.FULL

Jun Yina,b,*, Huili Xinga, and Jianping Yeb. "Efficacy of Berberine in Patients with Type-2 Diabetes," *Metabolism.* 2008 May ; 57(5): 712–717.

Kahn, C. R., Vicent, D. & Doria, A. "Genetics of non-insulin-dependent (type II) diabetes mellitus," *Annu. Rev. Med.* 47, 509–531 (1996).

Katahn, Martin. *The Rotation Diet,* W.W. Norton and Company, 1986

Kirchner, John. *Nutrition Almanac,* McGraw-Hill, 1973

Kirschmann, Gayla J. *Nutrition Almanac.* 4TH Ed. 1996

Kloss, Jethro. *Back to Eden,* Woodbridge Press Publishing Co., 1939, 1988

Kong WJ, Zhang H, Song DQ, Xue R, Zhao W, Wei J, Wang YM, Shan N, Zhou ZX, Yang P, You XF, Li ZR, Si SY, Zhao LX, Pan HN, Jiang JD. "Berberine reduces insulin resistance through protein kinase C-dependent up-regulation of insulin receptor expression," *Metabolism.* 2009 Jan;58(1):109–19.

Kopelman, P. G. "Obesity as a medical problem," *Nature* 404, 635–643 (2000).

Kubota, N. et al. "PPARg mediates high-fat diet-induced adipocyte hypertrophy and insulin resistance," *Mol. Cell* 4, 597–609 (1999).

Kunin, Richard A. *Mega-Nutrition,* McGraw-Hill Book Co., 1980

Kutsky, Roman J. *Handbook of Vitamins and Hormones,* Van Nostrand Reinhold Co., 1973

Lacey, Richard W. *Hard to Swallow: A Brief History of Food.* 1994

Lark, Susan M. MD, and Richards, James A., MBA. *The Chemistry of Success: Secrets of Peak Performance.* 2000

Lininger, Schuyler W, Jr. DC, editor-in-chief. *The Natural Pharmacy.* 1999

Macaulay VM. "Insulin-like growth factors and cancer," British Journal of Cancer 1992;65(3): 311–20.

Mazel, Judy. *The Beverly Hills Diet,* Macmillan Publishing Company, Inc., 1981

McCully. "Homocysteinemia and Arteriosclerosis," *American Heart Journal* 83:571–573, April, 1972

Merck Manual of Diagnosis and Therapy. 16TH Edition, 1992

Miles, P. D., Barak, Y., He, W., Evans, R. M. & Olefsky, J. M. "Improved insulin-sensitivity in mice heterozygous for PPAR-g deficiency," *J. Clin. Invest.* 105, 287–292 (2000).

Mohamed-Ali, V., Pinkney, J. H. & Coppack, S. W. Adipose tissue as an endocrine and paracrine organ. *Int. J. Obes. Relat. Metab. Disord.* 22, 1145–1158 (1998).

Moller, D. E. "Potential role of TNFa in the pathogenesis of insulin resistance and type-2 diabetes," *Trends Endocrinol. Metab.* 11, 212–217 (2000).

Morehouse, Lawrence E. and Gross, Leonard. *Total Fitness in 30 Minutes a Week,* Pocket Books, 1975

Morgan, Brian L.G. *Nutrition Prescription: Strategies for Preventing and Treating 50 Common Diseases,* Crown Publishers, Inc., 1987

Morgan, D. "Hormones May 'Program' Dieters' Weight Gain." CBS News Health Watch. September 10, 2010

Morley and Levine. "Stress Induced Eating is Mediated Through Endogenous Opiates," *Science* 209:1259–1260, 1980

Mortimore GE, Poso AR. "Intracellular protein catabolism and its control during nutrient deprivation and supply," *Annu Rev Nutr,* 1987;7:539

Mowbray, Scott. *The Food Fight.* 1992

Mukherjee, R. et al. "Sensitization of diabetic and obese mice to insulin by retinoid X receptor agonists," *Nature* 386, 407–410 (1997).

Munro, H.N. *Mammalian Protein Metabolism.* 1970.

Nestle, Marion. *Food Politics.* 2002

Newstrom, Harvey. *Nutrients Catalog.* 1993

Nilsson, Lennart. *The Body Victorious.* 1987

Novarra, Tova and Lipkowitz, Myron A. *Encyclopedia of Vitamins, Minerals, and Supplements.* 1996.

Orten, J.M. and Neuhaus, O.W. *Human Biochemistry,* 10TH edition, The C.V. Mosby Co., 1982

Palmer, S. and Bakshi, K. "Diet, Nutrition, and Cancer." *Journal of National Cancer Institute,* 70:1151–70, 1983

Pao, E. M., and Mickle, S.J. "Protein Nutrients in the United States." *Food Technology* 35:58–69, 1981

Passwater, Richard A. *Super Nutrition,* Pocket Books, 1975

Pearson, Durk and Shaw, Sandy. *Life Extension: A Practical Scientific Approach,* Warner Books, Inc., 1982

————. *Life Extension Companion,* Warner Books, Inc., 1984

————. *Life Extension Weight Loss Program,* Doubleday and Company, 1986

Pelstring, Linda, and Hauck, JoAnn. *Food to Improve Your Health.* 1974

Pennington, Jean A.T. and Church, Helen Nichols. *Food Values: of Portions Commonly Used,* Harper and Row, 1985

Phillips, R. L., and Snowdon, D. A. "Association of Meat and Coffee Use with Cancers of the Large Bowel, Breast, and Prostate Among Seventh Day Adventists: Preliminary Results." *Cancer Research Supplement,* 43:2403s–2408s, 1981

Physician's Desk Reference, 38th edition, Medical Economics Co., 1984

Pinckney and Pinckney. *The Encyclopedia of Medical Tests,* Pocket Books, 1978

Prevention Magazine's Complete Book of Vitamins, Rodale Press, 1977

Raloff, Janet. "Heart Risks: This is Nutty," *Science News,* Vol. 142, No. 4, p. 52, 1992

Raloff, Janet. "Hearty Vitamins: Sparing Arteries with Megadose Supplements," *Science News,* Vol 142, No. 5, p. 76, 1992

Raloff, Janet. "Teasing Out Dietary Cholesterol's Impact," *Science News,* Vol 141, No. 24, p. 390

Rayasam GV, et al. "Identification of berberine as a novel agonist of fatty acid receptor GPR40," *Phytother Res.* 2010 Aug;24(8):1260–3.

Reddy, B. S. "Dietary Factors and Cancer of the Large Bowel," *Semin Oncology* 3:351, 1976

Remington, Dennis and Fisher, Garth and Parent, Edward. *How to Lower Your Fat Thermostat,* Vitality House International, Inc., 1982

Reseland, Janne E. "Effect of long-term changes in diet and exercise on plasma leptin concentrations," *American Journal of Clinical Nutrition* Feb. 2001;73(2): 240–245

Rindos D. *The Origins of Agriculture: An Evolutionary Perspective.* Academic Press, 1987.

Robinson, Corinne H., MS, DSc (Hon), RD; Lawler, Marilyn R., MS, PhD, RD; Chenoweth, Wanda L.; MS, PhD, RD; and Garwick, Ann E., MS, RN. *Normal and Therapeutic Nutrition.* 17TH Edition. 1986

Ronzio, Robert A. *Encyclopedia of Nutrition and Good Health.* 1997

Rubin R, Baserga R. "Insulin-like growth factor-I receptor: Its role in cell proliferation, apoptosis, and tumorigenicity," Laboratory investigation; a journal of technical methods and pathology 1995;73(3): 311–31.

Ruby BC, Gaskill SE, Slivka D, Harger SG. "The addition of fenugreek extract *(Trigonella foenum-graecum)* to glucose feeding increases muscle glycogen resynthesis after exercise" *Amino Acids.* 2005 Feb;28(1):71–6. Epub 2004 Dec 2.

Rudin, Donald, MD, and Felix, Clara. *Omega-3 Oils.* 1996.

Schwartz, Bob. *Diets Don't Work,* Breakthru Publishing, 1982

Sears, Barry. *The Zone,* New York: HarperCollins Publishers, 1995

Shapiro, A., Mu, W., Roncal, C., et al, "Fructose-induced leptin resistance exacerbates weight gain in response to subsequent high-fat feeding," *Am. J. Physiol. Regul. Integr. Comp. Physiol.* Nov. 2008; 295 (5)

Shimomura, I., Hammer, R. E., Ikemoto, S., Brown, M. S. & Goldstein, J. L. "Leptin reverses insulin–resistance and diabetes mellitus in mice with congenital lipodystrophy," *Nature* 401, 73–76 (1999).

Smolin, Lori A., PhD, and Grosvenor, Mary B., MS, RD. *Nutrition: Science and Applications.* 2000

Sonberg, Lynn. *A-Z Guide to Toxic Foods and How to Avoid Them.* 1992

Spiegelman, B. M. & Flier, J. S. "Adipogenesis and obesity: rounding out the big picture," *Cell* 87, 377–389 (1996).

Stauber, John C., and Rampton, Sheldon. *Toxic Sludge is Good For You: Lies, Damn Lies and the Public Relations Industry.* 1995. *Stedman's Medical Dictionary, 26TH edition.* 1995

Steincrohn, Peter J. *Low Blood Sugar,* Signet Books, 1972

Steppan, C. M. et al. "A family of tissue-specific resistin-like molecules," *Proc. Natl Acad. Sci.* USA

Tappel. "Biological Antioxidant Protection Against Lipid Peroxidation Damage," *American Journal of Clinical Nutrition,* 23(8):1137–1139, 1970

Tontonoz, P., Hu, E. & Spiegelman, B. M. "Stimulation of adipogenesis in fibroblasts by PPARg2, a lipid-activated transcription factor," *Cell* 79, 1147–1156 (1994).

Tortora, Gerald J., and Anagnostakos, Nicholas P. *Principles of Anatomy and Physiology.* 5TH Edition. New York: Harper and Row, 1987

Tver, David F. and Russell, Percy, PhD. *The Nutrition and Health Encyclopedia.* 2ND Edition. 1989.

Ulene, Art, MD. *Dr. Art Ulene's Complete Guide to Vitamins, Minerals, and Herbs.* 2000

VanHeek, M. et al. "Diet-induced obese mice develop peripheral, but not central, resistance to leptin," *J. Clin. Invest.* 99, 385–390 (1997).

Visek, W. J. "Ammonia Metabolism, Urea Cycle Capacity, and Their Biochemical Assessment." *Nutrition Review,* 37(9):273–282, 1979

Whitney, Eleanor Noss and Hamilton, Eva May Nunnelley. *Understanding Nutrition,* West publishing Company, 1981

Wiggins P.M. "A Mechanism of ATP-Driven Cation Pumps"; PP-266–269, *Biophysics of Water*, Eds. Felix Franks and Sheila F. Mathis, John Wiley and Sons, Ltd. 1982

Willett, Walter C. MD. *Eat, Drink, and Be Healthy*. 2001

Williams, Roger J. *Nutrition Against Disease*, Bantam Books, 1971

Wolman, Benjamin B. *Psychological Aspects of Obesity*, Van Nostrand Reinhold, 1982

Wynder, E. L., et al. "Diet and Cancer of the Gastrointestinal Tract," *Adr. Internal Medicine*. 1977; 22:397–419.

Young VR, Bier DM, Pellett PL. "A theoretical basis for increasing current estimates of the amino acid requirements in adult man with experimental support," *Am J Clin Nutr*, 1989;50:80

Young, V. "Soy Protein in Relation to Human Protein and Amino Acid Nutrition." *Journal of American Dietetic Association*, 1991, 19:828–835.

Yudkin, J. "Dietary Factors in Atherosclerosis": Sugar, *Lipids*, 13:370–372, 1980

Zhang H, Wei J, Xue R, Wu JD, Zhao W, Wang ZZ, Wang SK, Zhou ZX, Song DQ, Wang YM, Pan HN, Kong WJ, Jiang JD. "Berberine lowers blood glucose in type 2 diabetes mellitus patients through increasing insulin receptor expression," *Metabolism*. 2010 Feb;59(2):285–92.

Ziegler, Ekhard E., and Filer, L.J. Jr., editors. *Present Knowledge in Nutrition*. 7TH Edition. 1996

NOTES

_____

_____

_____

_____

_____

_____

_____

_____

_____

_____

_____

_____

_____

_____

_____

_____

www.ingramcontent.com/pod-product-compliance
Lightning Source LLC
Chambersburg PA
CBHW060808270326
41928CB00002B/24